ECHOES OF THE QUIET HOUSE

THE HOUSE THAT WATCHES

It knows who's looking.

ROBERT ARMSTRONG

Ordering Information:
Quantity Sales: Special discounts are available for quantity purchases by corporations, associations, and others.
For details, contact the publisher at:
Email: contact@libraryusergroup.com

For orders from U.S. trade bookstores and wholesalers, please contact your distribution channel.

ISBN: 978-1-63553-030-8

Ebook: 978-1-63553-038-4

The Quiet House

The House That Watches

The main category of the book - Drama

First Edition

The footprint was still there in the morning, and somehow that made it worse.

Diana stood in the upstairs hallway of the blue house with her arms folded tight across her chest, staring at the single bare impression in the dust. It had formed the night before while she and Christopher were watching. Neither of them had touched the floor. Neither of them had moved close enough to disturb the dust.

Yet the print remained.

Too clear. Too deliberate.

Christopher crouched beside it again, camera in hand, his movements steady but more controlled than calm. "It should have softened overnight," he said quietly. "Dust doesn't hold edges like this unless something refreshes it."

Bosco gave a low warning rumble behind them.

Lilly sat halfway up the stairs, staring not at the print… but at the ceiling above it.

That was new.

Christopher noticed too. His flashlight slowly lifted upward, beam sliding across insulation and beams until it caught on a narrow seam running along the upper framing.

"…that wasn't there yesterday," he whispered.

Diana felt the first real chill of Book Two settle into her bones.

Because something in the house was no longer just reacting.

It was adjusting.

The house did not feel empty anymore. The silence behaved differently now, collecting in the corners and pressing softly against every small sound. Christopher noticed it every time he stepped inside. Diana felt it even more. Bosco tracked it with low warning rumbles, and Lilly watched the ceilings and vents as if expecting something to move when no one was looking.

The house did not feel empty anymore. The silence behaved differently now, collecting in the corners and pressing softly against every small sound. Christopher noticed it every time he stepped inside. Diana felt it even more. Bosco tracked it with low warning rumbles, and Lilly watched the ceilings and vents as if expecting something to move when no one was looking.

The house did not feel empty anymore. The silence behaved differently now, collecting in the corners and pressing softly against every small sound. Christopher noticed it every time he stepped inside. Diana felt it even more. Bosco tracked it with low warning rumbles, and Lilly watched the ceilings and vents as if expecting something to move when no one was looking.

The house did not feel empty anymore. The silence behaved differently now, collecting in the corners and pressing softly against every small sound. Christopher noticed it every time he stepped inside. Diana felt it even more. Bosco tracked it with low warning rumbles, and Lilly watched the ceilings and vents as if expecting something to move when no one was looking.

The house did not feel empty anymore. The silence behaved differently now, collecting in the corners and pressing softly against every small sound. Christopher noticed it every time he stepped inside. Diana felt it even more. Bosco tracked it with low warning rumbles, and Lilly watched the ceilings and vents as if expecting something to move when no one was looking.

The house did not feel empty anymore. The silence behaved differently now, collecting in the corners and pressing softly against every small sound. Christopher noticed it every time he stepped inside. Diana felt it even more. Bosco tracked it with low warning rumbles, and Lilly watched the ceilings and vents as if expecting something to move when no one was looking.

The house did not feel empty anymore. The silence behaved differently now, collecting in the corners and pressing softly against every small sound. Christopher noticed it every time he stepped inside. Diana felt it even more. Bosco tracked it with low warning rumbles, and Lilly watched the ceilings and vents as if expecting something to move when no one was looking.

The house did not feel empty anymore. The silence behaved differently now, collecting in the corners and pressing softly against every small sound. Christopher noticed it every time he stepped inside. Diana felt it even more. Bosco tracked it with low warning rumbles, and Lilly watched the ceilings and vents as if expecting something to move when no one was looking.

The house did not feel empty anymore. The silence behaved differently now, collecting in the corners and pressing softly against every small sound. Christopher noticed it every time he stepped inside. Diana felt it even more. Bosco tracked it with low warning rumbles, and Lilly watched the ceilings and vents as if expecting something to move when no one was looking.

The house did not feel empty anymore. The silence behaved differently now, collecting in the corners and pressing softly against every small sound. Christopher noticed it every time he stepped inside. Diana felt it even more. Bosco tracked it with low warning rumbles, and Lilly watched the ceilings and vents as if expecting something to move when no one was looking.

The house did not feel empty anymore. The silence behaved differently now, collecting in the corners and pressing softly against every small sound. Christopher noticed it every time he stepped inside. Diana felt it even more. Bosco tracked it with low warning rumbles, and Lilly watched the ceilings and vents as if expecting something to move when no one was looking.

The house did not feel empty anymore. The silence behaved differently now, collecting in the corners and pressing softly against every small sound. Christopher noticed it every time he stepped inside. Diana felt it even more. Bosco tracked it with low warning rumbles, and Lilly watched the ceilings and vents as if expecting something to move when no one was looking.

The house did not feel empty anymore. The silence behaved differently now, collecting in the corners and pressing softly against every small sound. Christopher noticed it every time he stepped inside. Diana felt it even more. Bosco tracked it with low warning rumbles, and Lilly watched the ceilings and vents as if expecting something to move when no one was looking.

The house did not feel empty anymore. The silence behaved differently now, collecting in the corners and pressing softly against every small sound. Christopher noticed it every time he stepped inside. Diana felt it even more. Bosco tracked it with low warning rumbles, and Lilly watched the ceilings and vents as if expecting something to move when no one was looking.

The house did not feel empty anymore. The silence behaved differently now, collecting in the corners and pressing softly against every small sound. Christopher noticed it every time he stepped inside. Diana felt it even more. Bosco tracked it with low warning rumbles, and Lilly watched the ceilings and vents as if expecting something to move when no one was looking.

Christopher spent most of the morning mapping the hidden spaces again, but the measurements refused to cooperate. The distances were slightly off—only inches at a time—but enough to make his jaw tighten.

"Walls don't drift," he muttered.

But Diana was no longer convinced the house was following normal rules.

By afternoon, Bosco refused to enter the hallway entirely. He planted himself near the foyer, muscles rigid, eyes locked toward the interior of the house.

Lilly had moved her attention to the vents.

Every few minutes, her ears twitched upward as if she were listening to movement traveling through the structure.

When the first soft thump came from somewhere inside the ceiling cavity, all three of them
heard it.

Christopher froze mid-measurement.

Diana's pulse jumped.

Because this time…

The sound clearly moved from one end of the
house to the other.

The house did not feel empty anymore. The
silence behaved differently now, collecting in the
corners and pressing softly against every small
sound. Christopher noticed it every time he
stepped inside. Diana felt it even more. Bosco
tracked it with low warning rumbles, and Lilly
watched the ceilings and vents as if expecting
something to move when no one was looking.

The house did not feel empty anymore. The silence behaved differently now, collecting in the corners and pressing softly against every small sound. Christopher noticed it every time he stepped inside. Diana felt it even more. Bosco tracked it with low warning rumbles, and Lilly watched the ceilings and vents as if expecting something to move when no one was looking.

The house did not feel empty anymore. The silence behaved differently now, collecting in the corners and pressing softly against every small sound. Christopher noticed it every time he stepped inside. Diana felt it even more. Bosco tracked it with low warning rumbles, and Lilly watched the ceilings and vents as if expecting something to move when no one was looking.

The house did not feel empty anymore. The silence behaved differently now, collecting in the corners and pressing softly against every small sound. Christopher noticed it every time he stepped inside. Diana felt it even more. Bosco tracked it with low warning rumbles, and Lilly watched the ceilings and vents as if expecting something to move when no one was looking.

The house did not feel empty anymore. The silence behaved differently now, collecting in the corners and pressing softly against every small sound. Christopher noticed it every time he stepped inside. Diana felt it even more. Bosco tracked it with low warning rumbles, and Lilly watched the ceilings and vents as if expecting something to move when no one was looking.

The house did not feel empty anymore. The silence behaved differently now, collecting in the corners and pressing softly against every small sound. Christopher noticed it every time he stepped inside. Diana felt it even more. Bosco tracked it with low warning rumbles, and Lilly watched the ceilings and vents as if expecting something to move when no one was looking.

The house did not feel empty anymore. The silence behaved differently now, collecting in the corners and pressing softly against every small sound. Christopher noticed it every time he stepped inside. Diana felt it even more. Bosco tracked it with low warning rumbles, and Lilly watched the ceilings and vents as if expecting something to move when no one was looking.

The house did not feel empty anymore. The silence behaved differently now, collecting in the corners and pressing softly against every small sound. Christopher noticed it every time he stepped inside. Diana felt it even more. Bosco tracked it with low warning rumbles, and Lilly watched the ceilings and vents as if expecting something to move when no one was looking.

The house did not feel empty anymore. The silence behaved differently now, collecting in the corners and pressing softly against every small sound. Christopher noticed it every time he stepped inside. Diana felt it even more. Bosco tracked it with low warning rumbles, and Lilly watched the ceilings and vents as if expecting something to move when no one was looking.

The house did not feel empty anymore. The silence behaved differently now, collecting in the corners and pressing softly against every small sound. Christopher noticed it every time he stepped inside. Diana felt it even more. Bosco tracked it with low warning rumbles, and Lilly watched the ceilings and vents as if expecting something to move when no one was looking.

The house did not feel empty anymore. The silence behaved differently now, collecting in the corners and pressing softly against every small sound. Christopher noticed it every time he stepped inside. Diana felt it even more. Bosco tracked it with low warning rumbles, and Lilly watched the ceilings and vents as if expecting something to move when no one was looking.

The house did not feel empty anymore. The silence behaved differently now, collecting in the corners and pressing softly against every small sound. Christopher noticed it every time he stepped inside. Diana felt it even more. Bosco tracked it with low warning rumbles, and Lilly watched the ceilings and vents as if expecting something to move when no one was looking.

The house did not feel empty anymore. The silence behaved differently now, collecting in the corners and pressing softly against every small sound. Christopher noticed it every time he stepped inside. Diana felt it even more. Bosco tracked it with low warning rumbles, and Lilly watched the ceilings and vents as if expecting something to move when no one was looking.

The house did not feel empty anymore. The silence behaved differently now, collecting in the corners and pressing softly against every small sound. Christopher noticed it every time he stepped inside. Diana felt it even more. Bosco tracked it with low warning rumbles, and Lilly watched the ceilings and vents as if expecting something to move when no one was looking.

The house did not feel empty anymore. The silence behaved differently now, collecting in the corners and pressing softly against every small sound. Christopher noticed it every time he stepped inside. Diana felt it even more. Bosco tracked it with low warning rumbles, and Lilly watched the ceilings and vents as if expecting something to move when no one was looking.

The house did not feel empty anymore. The silence behaved differently now, collecting in the corners and pressing softly against every small sound. Christopher noticed it every time he stepped inside. Diana felt it even more. Bosco tracked it with low warning rumbles, and Lilly watched the ceilings and vents as if expecting something to move when no one was looking.

The updated blueprint made things worse.

Christopher spread the new measurements across Diana's kitchen table, drawing lines with tight, precise movements. "These spaces shouldn't connect like this," he said.

But they did.

The hidden cavities formed a loose loop through the structure—one that did not appear on any original plans.

Lenny studied the map longer than either of them.

"That's not renovation work," he said finally. "That's long-term modification."

Diana looked up sharply. "You mean someone built this on purpose?"

Lenny's expression was unreadable.

"I mean," he said slowly, "someone wanted movement inside these walls."

That night, the upstairs camera glitched for exactly seven seconds.

When it came back online…

The hallway dust had been disturbed again.

The house did not feel empty anymore. The silence behaved differently now, collecting in the corners and pressing softly against every small sound. Christopher noticed it every time he stepped inside. Diana felt it even more. Bosco tracked it with low warning rumbles, and Lilly watched the ceilings and vents as if expecting

something to move when no one was looking.

The house did not feel empty anymore. The silence behaved differently now, collecting in the corners and pressing softly against every small sound. Christopher noticed it every time he stepped inside. Diana felt it even more. Bosco tracked it with low warning rumbles, and Lilly watched the ceilings and vents as if expecting something to move when no one was looking.

The house did not feel empty anymore. The silence behaved differently now, collecting in the corners and pressing softly against every small sound. Christopher noticed it every time he stepped inside. Diana felt it even more. Bosco tracked it with low warning rumbles, and Lilly watched the ceilings and vents as if expecting something to move when no one was looking.

The house did not feel empty anymore. The silence behaved differently now, collecting in the corners and pressing softly against every small sound. Christopher noticed it every time he stepped inside. Diana felt it even more. Bosco tracked it with low warning rumbles, and Lilly watched the ceilings and vents as if expecting

something to move when no one was looking.

The house did not feel empty anymore. The silence behaved differently now, collecting in the corners and pressing softly against every small sound. Christopher noticed it every time he stepped inside. Diana felt it even more. Bosco tracked it with low warning rumbles, and Lilly watched the ceilings and vents as if expecting something to move when no one was looking.

The house did not feel empty anymore. The silence behaved differently now, collecting in the corners and pressing softly against every small sound. Christopher noticed it every time he stepped inside. Diana felt it even more. Bosco tracked it with low warning rumbles, and Lilly watched the ceilings and vents as if expecting something to move when no one was looking.

The house did not feel empty anymore. The silence behaved differently now, collecting in the corners and pressing softly against every small sound. Christopher noticed it every time he stepped inside. Diana felt it even more. Bosco tracked it with low warning rumbles, and Lilly watched the ceilings and vents as if expecting

something to move when no one was looking.

The house did not feel empty anymore. The silence behaved differently now, collecting in the corners and pressing softly against every small sound. Christopher noticed it every time he stepped inside. Diana felt it even more. Bosco tracked it with low warning rumbles, and Lilly watched the ceilings and vents as if expecting something to move when no one was looking.

The house did not feel empty anymore. The silence behaved differently now, collecting in the corners and pressing softly against every small sound. Christopher noticed it every time he stepped inside. Diana felt it even more. Bosco tracked it with low warning rumbles, and Lilly watched the ceilings and vents as if expecting something to move when no one was looking.

The house did not feel empty anymore. The silence behaved differently now, collecting in the corners and pressing softly against every small sound. Christopher noticed it every time he stepped inside. Diana felt it even more. Bosco tracked it with low warning rumbles, and Lilly watched the ceilings and vents as if expecting

something to move when no one was looking.

The house did not feel empty anymore. The silence behaved differently now, collecting in the corners and pressing softly against every small sound. Christopher noticed it every time he stepped inside. Diana felt it even more. Bosco tracked it with low warning rumbles, and Lilly watched the ceilings and vents as if expecting something to move when no one was looking.

The house did not feel empty anymore. The silence behaved differently now, collecting in the corners and pressing softly against every small sound. Christopher noticed it every time he stepped inside. Diana felt it even more. Bosco tracked it with low warning rumbles, and Lilly watched the ceilings and vents as if expecting something to move when no one was looking.

The house did not feel empty anymore. The silence behaved differently now, collecting in the corners and pressing softly against every small sound. Christopher noticed it every time he stepped inside. Diana felt it even more. Bosco tracked it with low warning rumbles, and Lilly watched the ceilings and vents as if expecting

something to move when no one was looking.

The house did not feel empty anymore. The silence behaved differently now, collecting in the corners and pressing softly against every small sound. Christopher noticed it every time he stepped inside. Diana felt it even more. Bosco tracked it with low warning rumbles, and Lilly watched the ceilings and vents as if expecting something to move when no one was looking.

The house did not feel empty anymore. The silence behaved differently now, collecting in the corners and pressing softly against every small sound. Christopher noticed it every time he stepped inside. Diana felt it even more. Bosco tracked it with low warning rumbles, and Lilly watched the ceilings and vents as if expecting something to move when no one was looking.

The house did not feel empty anymore. The silence behaved differently now, collecting in the corners and pressing softly against every small sound. Christopher noticed it every time he stepped inside. Diana felt it even more. Bosco tracked it with low warning rumbles, and Lilly watched the ceilings and vents as if expecting

something to move when no one was looking.

The house did not feel empty anymore. The silence behaved differently now, collecting in the corners and pressing softly against every small sound. Christopher noticed it every time he stepped inside. Diana felt it even more. Bosco tracked it with low warning rumbles, and Lilly watched the ceilings and vents as if expecting something to move when no one was looking.

They added more cameras.

Christopher installed them himself—hallway, passage entrance, second-floor landing. He triple-checked the wiring like a man who trusted equipment more than instincts.

At 2:14 a.m., the first anomaly appeared.

Not movement.

Not clearly.

But the camera time stamp skipped backward three seconds… then forward again.

Diana replayed the clip twice.

Christopher watched it five times.

Bosco began growling before the next glitch even started.

And Lilly—silent, still—turned slowly to stare directly into the nearest camera lens.

As if something behind it had just moved.

The house did not feel empty anymore. The silence behaved differently now, collecting in the corners and pressing softly against every small sound. Christopher noticed it every time he stepped inside. Diana felt it even more. Bosco tracked it with low warning rumbles, and Lilly watched the ceilings and vents as if expecting something to move when no one was looking.

The house did not feel empty anymore. The silence behaved differently now, collecting in the corners and pressing softly against every small sound. Christopher noticed it every time he stepped inside. Diana felt it even more. Bosco

tracked it with low warning rumbles, and Lilly watched the ceilings and vents as if expecting something to move when no one was looking.

The house did not feel empty anymore. The silence behaved differently now, collecting in the corners and pressing softly against every small sound. Christopher noticed it every time he stepped inside. Diana felt it even more. Bosco tracked it with low warning rumbles, and Lilly watched the ceilings and vents as if expecting something to move when no one was looking.

The house did not feel empty anymore. The silence behaved differently now, collecting in the corners and pressing softly against every small sound. Christopher noticed it every time he stepped inside. Diana felt it even more. Bosco tracked it with low warning rumbles, and Lilly watched the ceilings and vents as if expecting something to move when no one was looking.

The house did not feel empty anymore. The silence behaved differently now, collecting in the corners and pressing softly against every small sound. Christopher noticed it every time he stepped inside. Diana felt it even more. Bosco

tracked it with low warning rumbles, and Lilly watched the ceilings and vents as if expecting something to move when no one was looking.

The house did not feel empty anymore. The silence behaved differently now, collecting in the corners and pressing softly against every small sound. Christopher noticed it every time he stepped inside. Diana felt it even more. Bosco tracked it with low warning rumbles, and Lilly watched the ceilings and vents as if expecting something to move when no one was looking.

The house did not feel empty anymore. The silence behaved differently now, collecting in the corners and pressing softly against every small sound. Christopher noticed it every time he stepped inside. Diana felt it even more. Bosco tracked it with low warning rumbles, and Lilly watched the ceilings and vents as if expecting something to move when no one was looking.

The house did not feel empty anymore. The silence behaved differently now, collecting in the corners and pressing softly against every small sound. Christopher noticed it every time he stepped inside. Diana felt it even more. Bosco

tracked it with low warning rumbles, and Lilly watched the ceilings and vents as if expecting something to move when no one was looking.

The house did not feel empty anymore. The silence behaved differently now, collecting in the corners and pressing softly against every small sound. Christopher noticed it every time he stepped inside. Diana felt it even more. Bosco tracked it with low warning rumbles, and Lilly watched the ceilings and vents as if expecting something to move when no one was looking.

The house did not feel empty anymore. The silence behaved differently now, collecting in the corners and pressing softly against every small sound. Christopher noticed it every time he stepped inside. Diana felt it even more. Bosco tracked it with low warning rumbles, and Lilly watched the ceilings and vents as if expecting something to move when no one was looking.

The house did not feel empty anymore. The silence behaved differently now, collecting in the corners and pressing softly against every small sound. Christopher noticed it every time he stepped inside. Diana felt it even more. Bosco

tracked it with low warning rumbles, and Lilly watched the ceilings and vents as if expecting something to move when no one was looking.

The house did not feel empty anymore. The silence behaved differently now, collecting in the corners and pressing softly against every small sound. Christopher noticed it every time he stepped inside. Diana felt it even more. Bosco tracked it with low warning rumbles, and Lilly watched the ceilings and vents as if expecting something to move when no one was looking.

The house did not feel empty anymore. The silence behaved differently now, collecting in the corners and pressing softly against every small sound. Christopher noticed it every time he stepped inside. Diana felt it even more. Bosco tracked it with low warning rumbles, and Lilly watched the ceilings and vents as if expecting something to move when no one was looking.

The house did not feel empty anymore. The silence behaved differently now, collecting in the corners and pressing softly against every small sound. Christopher noticed it every time he stepped inside. Diana felt it even more. Bosco

tracked it with low warning rumbles, and Lilly watched the ceilings and vents as if expecting something to move when no one was looking.

The house did not feel empty anymore. The silence behaved differently now, collecting in the corners and pressing softly against every small sound. Christopher noticed it every time he stepped inside. Diana felt it even more. Bosco tracked it with low warning rumbles, and Lilly watched the ceilings and vents as if expecting something to move when no one was looking.

The house did not feel empty anymore. The silence behaved differently now, collecting in the corners and pressing softly against every small sound. Christopher noticed it every time he stepped inside. Diana felt it even more. Bosco tracked it with low warning rumbles, and Lilly watched the ceilings and vents as if expecting something to move when no one was looking.

The house did not feel empty anymore. The silence behaved differently now, collecting in the corners and pressing softly against every small sound. Christopher noticed it every time he stepped inside. Diana felt it even more. Bosco

tracked it with low warning rumbles, and Lilly watched the ceilings and vents as if expecting something to move when no one was looking.

The House That Watches — Chapter 5: Lenny's Half-Truth

Diana found Lenny at The Blue Jay again, exactly where he always seemed to be when things escalated.

"You're digging deeper," he said before she even sat down.

She didn't bother denying it.

When she described the expanding passages, Lenny's humor faded for the first time.

"The Keller disappearance in '65," he said quietly, "wasn't the only strange thing about that house."

Diana leaned forward. "What else happened?"

Lenny hesitated—a rare crack in his usual rhythm.

"People used to complain," he said slowly. "Said the house made them feel… observed."

A cold weight settled in Diana's stomach.

Because across the street…

The upstairs light of the blue house flicked on by itself.

And this time—

It stayed on.

The house did not feel empty anymore. The silence behaved differently now, collecting in the corners and pressing softly against every small sound. Christopher noticed it every time he stepped inside. Diana felt it even more. Bosco tracked it with low warning rumbles, and Lilly watched the ceilings and vents as if expecting

something to move when no one was looking.

The house did not feel empty anymore. The silence behaved differently now, collecting in the corners and pressing softly against every small sound. Christopher noticed it every time he stepped inside. Diana felt it even more. Bosco tracked it with low warning rumbles, and Lilly watched the ceilings and vents as if expecting something to move when no one was looking.

The house did not feel empty anymore. The silence behaved differently now, collecting in the corners and pressing softly against every small sound. Christopher noticed it every time he stepped inside. Diana felt it even more. Bosco tracked it with low warning rumbles, and Lilly watched the ceilings and vents as if expecting something to move when no one was looking.

The house did not feel empty anymore. The silence behaved differently now, collecting in the corners and pressing softly against every small sound. Christopher noticed it every time he stepped inside. Diana felt it even more. Bosco tracked it with low warning rumbles, and Lilly watched the ceilings and vents as if expecting

something to move when no one was looking.

The house did not feel empty anymore. The silence behaved differently now, collecting in the corners and pressing softly against every small sound. Christopher noticed it every time he stepped inside. Diana felt it even more. Bosco tracked it with low warning rumbles, and Lilly watched the ceilings and vents as if expecting something to move when no one was looking.

The house did not feel empty anymore. The silence behaved differently now, collecting in the corners and pressing softly against every small sound. Christopher noticed it every time he stepped inside. Diana felt it even more. Bosco tracked it with low warning rumbles, and Lilly watched the ceilings and vents as if expecting something to move when no one was looking.

The house did not feel empty anymore. The silence behaved differently now, collecting in the corners and pressing softly against every small sound. Christopher noticed it every time he stepped inside. Diana felt it even more. Bosco tracked it with low warning rumbles, and Lilly watched the ceilings and vents as if expecting

something to move when no one was looking.

The house did not feel empty anymore. The silence behaved differently now, collecting in the corners and pressing softly against every small sound. Christopher noticed it every time he stepped inside. Diana felt it even more. Bosco tracked it with low warning rumbles, and Lilly watched the ceilings and vents as if expecting something to move when no one was looking.

The house did not feel empty anymore. The silence behaved differently now, collecting in the corners and pressing softly against every small sound. Christopher noticed it every time he stepped inside. Diana felt it even more. Bosco tracked it with low warning rumbles, and Lilly watched the ceilings and vents as if expecting something to move when no one was looking.

The house did not feel empty anymore. The silence behaved differently now, collecting in the corners and pressing softly against every small sound. Christopher noticed it every time he stepped inside. Diana felt it even more. Bosco tracked it with low warning rumbles, and Lilly watched the ceilings and vents as if expecting

something to move when no one was looking.

The house did not feel empty anymore. The silence behaved differently now, collecting in the corners and pressing softly against every small sound. Christopher noticed it every time he stepped inside. Diana felt it even more. Bosco tracked it with low warning rumbles, and Lilly watched the ceilings and vents as if expecting something to move when no one was looking.

The house did not feel empty anymore. The silence behaved differently now, collecting in the corners and pressing softly against every small sound. Christopher noticed it every time he stepped inside. Diana felt it even more. Bosco tracked it with low warning rumbles, and Lilly watched the ceilings and vents as if expecting something to move when no one was looking.

The house did not feel empty anymore. The silence behaved differently now, collecting in the corners and pressing softly against every small sound. Christopher noticed it every time he stepped inside. Diana felt it even more. Bosco tracked it with low warning rumbles, and Lilly watched the ceilings and vents as if expecting

something to move when no one was looking.

The house did not feel empty anymore. The silence behaved differently now, collecting in the corners and pressing softly against every small sound. Christopher noticed it every time he stepped inside. Diana felt it even more. Bosco tracked it with low warning rumbles, and Lilly watched the ceilings and vents as if expecting something to move when no one was looking.

The house did not feel empty anymore. The silence behaved differently now, collecting in the corners and pressing softly against every small sound. Christopher noticed it every time he stepped inside. Diana felt it even more. Bosco tracked it with low warning rumbles, and Lilly watched the ceilings and vents as if expecting something to move when no one was looking.

The house did not feel empty anymore. The silence behaved differently now, collecting in the corners and pressing softly against every small sound. Christopher noticed it every time he stepped inside. Diana felt it even more. Bosco tracked it with low warning rumbles, and Lilly watched the ceilings and vents as if expecting

something to move when no one was looking.

The house did not feel empty anymore. The silence behaved differently now, collecting in the corners and pressing softly against every small sound. Christopher noticed it every time he stepped inside. Diana felt it even more. Bosco tracked it with low warning rumbles, and Lilly watched the ceilings and vents as if expecting something to move when no one was looking.

Christopher ran the thermal scanner three times before he said anything.

The readings didn't make sense.

Cold pockets had formed inside the blue house—tight, contained zones where the temperature dropped nearly ten degrees in precise oval shapes along the walls. Not random. Not draft-related.

Patterned.

Diana watched the screen over his shoulder. "HVAC issue?"

Christopher didn't answer right away.

Because the cold zones were moving.

Slowly.

Measured.

Tracking the same path the footprints had followed days earlier.

Bosco began growling before the scanner even
finished updating.

And Lilly—perfectly still—turned her head in
slow unison with the shifting cold spot.

As if she could see it without the machine.

The house felt more aware with each passing
hour. The quiet gathered along the walls and
ceilings as if it were listening back. Christopher
noticed the change immediately. Diana felt it in
the pit of her stomach. Bosco tracked it with low
warning rumbles, and Lilly stared into empty

spaces with unsettling patience.

The house felt more aware with each passing hour. The quiet gathered along the walls and ceilings as if it were listening back. Christopher noticed the change immediately. Diana felt it in the pit of her stomach. Bosco tracked it with low warning rumbles, and Lilly stared into empty spaces with unsettling patience.

The house felt more aware with each passing hour. The quiet gathered along the walls and ceilings as if it were listening back. Christopher noticed the change immediately. Diana felt it in the pit of her stomach. Bosco tracked it with low warning rumbles, and Lilly stared into empty spaces with unsettling patience.

The house felt more aware with each passing hour. The quiet gathered along the walls and ceilings as if it were listening back. Christopher noticed the change immediately. Diana felt it in the pit of her stomach. Bosco tracked it with low warning rumbles, and Lilly stared into empty spaces with unsettling patience.

The house felt more aware with each passing hour. The quiet gathered along the walls and ceilings as if it were listening back. Christopher noticed the change immediately. Diana felt it in the pit of her stomach. Bosco tracked it with low warning rumbles, and Lilly stared into empty spaces with unsettling patience.

The house felt more aware with each passing hour. The quiet gathered along the walls and ceilings as if it were listening back. Christopher noticed the change immediately. Diana felt it in the pit of her stomach. Bosco tracked it with low warning rumbles, and Lilly stared into empty spaces with unsettling patience.

The house felt more aware with each passing hour. The quiet gathered along the walls and ceilings as if it were listening back. Christopher noticed the change immediately. Diana felt it in the pit of her stomach. Bosco tracked it with low warning rumbles, and Lilly stared into empty spaces with unsettling patience.

The house felt more aware with each passing hour. The quiet gathered along the walls and ceilings as if it were listening back. Christopher

noticed the change immediately. Diana felt it in the pit of her stomach. Bosco tracked it with low warning rumbles, and Lilly stared into empty spaces with unsettling patience.

The house felt more aware with each passing hour. The quiet gathered along the walls and ceilings as if it were listening back. Christopher noticed the change immediately. Diana felt it in the pit of her stomach. Bosco tracked it with low warning rumbles, and Lilly stared into empty spaces with unsettling patience.

The house felt more aware with each passing hour. The quiet gathered along the walls and ceilings as if it were listening back. Christopher noticed the change immediately. Diana felt it in the pit of her stomach. Bosco tracked it with low warning rumbles, and Lilly stared into empty spaces with unsettling patience.

The house felt more aware with each passing hour. The quiet gathered along the walls and ceilings as if it were listening back. Christopher noticed the change immediately. Diana felt it in the pit of her stomach. Bosco tracked it with low warning rumbles, and Lilly stared into empty

spaces with unsettling patience.

The house felt more aware with each passing hour. The quiet gathered along the walls and ceilings as if it were listening back. Christopher noticed the change immediately. Diana felt it in the pit of her stomach. Bosco tracked it with low warning rumbles, and Lilly stared into empty spaces with unsettling patience.

The house felt more aware with each passing hour. The quiet gathered along the walls and ceilings as if it were listening back. Christopher noticed the change immediately. Diana felt it in the pit of her stomach. Bosco tracked it with low warning rumbles, and Lilly stared into empty spaces with unsettling patience.

The house felt more aware with each passing hour. The quiet gathered along the walls and ceilings as if it were listening back. Christopher noticed the change immediately. Diana felt it in the pit of her stomach. Bosco tracked it with low warning rumbles, and Lilly stared into empty spaces with unsettling patience.

The house felt more aware with each passing hour. The quiet gathered along the walls and ceilings as if it were listening back. Christopher noticed the change immediately. Diana felt it in the pit of her stomach. Bosco tracked it with low warning rumbles, and Lilly stared into empty spaces with unsettling patience.

The house felt more aware with each passing hour. The quiet gathered along the walls and ceilings as if it were listening back. Christopher noticed the change immediately. Diana felt it in the pit of her stomach. Bosco tracked it with low warning rumbles, and Lilly stared into empty spaces with unsettling patience.

The house felt more aware with each passing hour. The quiet gathered along the walls and ceilings as if it were listening back. Christopher noticed the change immediately. Diana felt it in the pit of her stomach. Bosco tracked it with low warning rumbles, and Lilly stared into empty spaces with unsettling patience.

The house felt more aware with each passing hour. The quiet gathered along the walls and ceilings as if it were listening back. Christopher

noticed the change immediately. Diana felt it in the pit of her stomach. Bosco tracked it with low warning rumbles, and Lilly stared into empty spaces with unsettling patience.

The house felt more aware with each passing hour. The quiet gathered along the walls and ceilings as if it were listening back. Christopher noticed the change immediately. Diana felt it in the pit of her stomach. Bosco tracked it with low warning rumbles, and Lilly stared into empty spaces with unsettling patience.

The deeper Christopher mapped, the worse it got.

Hidden framing extended beyond the original wall depth—older wood buried behind newer reinforcement. Someone hadn't just modified the house.

They had layered it.

Christopher crouched inside the passage, running his hand along the secondary studs. "This was done years apart," he said. "Different tools. Different materials."

Diana felt the weight of that settle heavily.

"How many times?" she asked.

Christopher didn't answer.

From somewhere above them, a slow dragging sound moved through the ceiling cavity.

Not quick.

Not random.

Traveling with purpose.

Bosco backed toward the doorway, ears pinned flat.

Because whatever was moving…

Was now directly overhead.

The house felt more aware with each passing hour. The quiet gathered along the walls and ceilings as if it were listening back. Christopher noticed the change immediately. Diana felt it in the pit of her stomach. Bosco tracked it with low warning rumbles, and Lilly stared into empty spaces with unsettling patience.

The house felt more aware with each passing hour. The quiet gathered along the walls and ceilings as if it were listening back. Christopher noticed the change immediately. Diana felt it in the pit of her stomach. Bosco tracked it with low warning rumbles, and Lilly stared into empty spaces with unsettling patience.

The house felt more aware with each passing hour. The quiet gathered along the walls and ceilings as if it were listening back. Christopher noticed the change immediately. Diana felt it in the pit of her stomach. Bosco tracked it with low warning rumbles, and Lilly stared into empty spaces with unsettling patience.

The house felt more aware with each passing hour. The quiet gathered along the walls and ceilings as if it were listening back. Christopher noticed the change immediately. Diana felt it in the pit of her stomach. Bosco tracked it with low warning rumbles, and Lilly stared into empty spaces with unsettling patience.

The house felt more aware with each passing hour. The quiet gathered along the walls and ceilings as if it were listening back. Christopher noticed the change immediately. Diana felt it in the pit of her stomach. Bosco tracked it with low warning rumbles, and Lilly stared into empty spaces with unsettling patience.

The house felt more aware with each passing hour. The quiet gathered along the walls and ceilings as if it were listening back. Christopher noticed the change immediately. Diana felt it in the pit of her stomach. Bosco tracked it with low warning rumbles, and Lilly stared into empty spaces with unsettling patience.

The house felt more aware with each passing hour. The quiet gathered along the walls and ceilings as if it were listening back. Christopher noticed the change immediately. Diana felt it in the pit of her stomach. Bosco tracked it with low warning rumbles, and Lilly stared into empty spaces with unsettling patience.

The house felt more aware with each passing hour. The quiet gathered along the walls and ceilings as if it were listening back. Christopher noticed the change immediately. Diana felt it in the pit of her stomach. Bosco tracked it with low warning rumbles, and Lilly stared into empty spaces with unsettling patience.

The house felt more aware with each passing hour. The quiet gathered along the walls and ceilings as if it were listening back. Christopher noticed the change immediately. Diana felt it in the pit of her stomach. Bosco tracked it with low warning rumbles, and Lilly stared into empty spaces with unsettling patience.

The house felt more aware with each passing hour. The quiet gathered along the walls and ceilings as if it were listening back. Christopher noticed the change immediately. Diana felt it in the pit of her stomach. Bosco tracked it with low warning rumbles, and Lilly stared into empty spaces with unsettling patience.

The house felt more aware with each passing

hour. The quiet gathered along the walls and ceilings as if it were listening back. Christopher noticed the change immediately. Diana felt it in the pit of her stomach. Bosco tracked it with low warning rumbles, and Lilly stared into empty spaces with unsettling patience.

The house felt more aware with each passing hour. The quiet gathered along the walls and ceilings as if it were listening back. Christopher noticed the change immediately. Diana felt it in the pit of her stomach. Bosco tracked it with low warning rumbles, and Lilly stared into empty spaces with unsettling patience.

The house felt more aware with each passing hour. The quiet gathered along the walls and ceilings as if it were listening back. Christopher noticed the change immediately. Diana felt it in the pit of her stomach. Bosco tracked it with low warning rumbles, and Lilly stared into empty spaces with unsettling patience.

The house felt more aware with each passing hour. The quiet gathered along the walls and ceilings as if it were listening back. Christopher noticed the change immediately. Diana felt it in

the pit of her stomach. Bosco tracked it with low warning rumbles, and Lilly stared into empty spaces with unsettling patience.

The house felt more aware with each passing hour. The quiet gathered along the walls and ceilings as if it were listening back. Christopher noticed the change immediately. Diana felt it in the pit of her stomach. Bosco tracked it with low warning rumbles, and Lilly stared into empty spaces with unsettling patience.

The house felt more aware with each passing hour. The quiet gathered along the walls and ceilings as if it were listening back. Christopher noticed the change immediately. Diana felt it in the pit of her stomach. Bosco tracked it with low warning rumbles, and Lilly stared into empty spaces with unsettling patience.

The house felt more aware with each passing hour. The quiet gathered along the walls and ceilings as if it were listening back. Christopher noticed the change immediately. Diana felt it in the pit of her stomach. Bosco tracked it with low warning rumbles, and Lilly stared into empty spaces with unsettling patience.

The house felt more aware with each passing hour. The quiet gathered along the walls and ceilings as if it were listening back. Christopher noticed the change immediately. Diana felt it in the pit of her stomach. Bosco tracked it with low warning rumbles, and Lilly stared into empty spaces with unsettling patience.

The house felt more aware with each passing hour. The quiet gathered along the walls and ceilings as if it were listening back. Christopher noticed the change immediately. Diana felt it in the pit of her stomach. Bosco tracked it with low warning rumbles, and Lilly stared into empty spaces with unsettling patience.

They stayed out of the house for exactly six hours.

When Christopher returned, one of the interior cameras was offline.

Not broken.

Disconnected.

The wiring hung loose from the wall exactly where he had secured it earlier that day.

Christopher stared at it for a long moment.

"I triple-checked this," he said quietly.

Diana didn't doubt him.

Because Bosco refused to cross the threshold at all now.

And Lilly sat in the foyer, staring up toward the second floor like something had just passed overhead.

Christopher reconnected the feed.

The missing footage covered nine minutes.

When playback resumed…

The hallway dust had been disturbed again.

The house felt more aware with each passing hour. The quiet gathered along the walls and ceilings as if it were listening back. Christopher noticed the change immediately. Diana felt it in the pit of her stomach. Bosco tracked it with low warning rumbles, and Lilly stared into empty

spaces with unsettling patience.

The house felt more aware with each passing hour. The quiet gathered along the walls and ceilings as if it were listening back. Christopher noticed the change immediately. Diana felt it in the pit of her stomach. Bosco tracked it with low warning rumbles, and Lilly stared into empty spaces with unsettling patience.

The house felt more aware with each passing hour. The quiet gathered along the walls and ceilings as if it were listening back. Christopher noticed the change immediately. Diana felt it in the pit of her stomach. Bosco tracked it with low warning rumbles, and Lilly stared into empty spaces with unsettling patience.

The house felt more aware with each passing hour. The quiet gathered along the walls and ceilings as if it were listening back. Christopher noticed the change immediately. Diana felt it in the pit of her stomach. Bosco tracked it with low warning rumbles, and Lilly stared into empty spaces with unsettling patience.

The house felt more aware with each passing hour. The quiet gathered along the walls and ceilings as if it were listening back. Christopher noticed the change immediately. Diana felt it in the pit of her stomach. Bosco tracked it with low warning rumbles, and Lilly stared into empty spaces with unsettling patience.

The house felt more aware with each passing hour. The quiet gathered along the walls and ceilings as if it were listening back. Christopher noticed the change immediately. Diana felt it in the pit of her stomach. Bosco tracked it with low warning rumbles, and Lilly stared into empty spaces with unsettling patience.

The house felt more aware with each passing hour. The quiet gathered along the walls and ceilings as if it were listening back. Christopher noticed the change immediately. Diana felt it in the pit of her stomach. Bosco tracked it with low warning rumbles, and Lilly stared into empty spaces with unsettling patience.

The house felt more aware with each passing hour. The quiet gathered along the walls and ceilings as if it were listening back. Christopher

noticed the change immediately. Diana felt it in the pit of her stomach. Bosco tracked it with low warning rumbles, and Lilly stared into empty spaces with unsettling patience.

The house felt more aware with each passing hour. The quiet gathered along the walls and ceilings as if it were listening back. Christopher noticed the change immediately. Diana felt it in the pit of her stomach. Bosco tracked it with low warning rumbles, and Lilly stared into empty spaces with unsettling patience.

The house felt more aware with each passing hour. The quiet gathered along the walls and ceilings as if it were listening back. Christopher noticed the change immediately. Diana felt it in the pit of her stomach. Bosco tracked it with low warning rumbles, and Lilly stared into empty spaces with unsettling patience.

The house felt more aware with each passing hour. The quiet gathered along the walls and ceilings as if it were listening back. Christopher noticed the change immediately. Diana felt it in the pit of her stomach. Bosco tracked it with low warning rumbles, and Lilly stared into empty

spaces with unsettling patience.

The house felt more aware with each passing hour. The quiet gathered along the walls and ceilings as if it were listening back. Christopher noticed the change immediately. Diana felt it in the pit of her stomach. Bosco tracked it with low warning rumbles, and Lilly stared into empty spaces with unsettling patience.

The house felt more aware with each passing hour. The quiet gathered along the walls and ceilings as if it were listening back. Christopher noticed the change immediately. Diana felt it in the pit of her stomach. Bosco tracked it with low warning rumbles, and Lilly stared into empty spaces with unsettling patience.

The house felt more aware with each passing hour. The quiet gathered along the walls and ceilings as if it were listening back. Christopher noticed the change immediately. Diana felt it in the pit of her stomach. Bosco tracked it with low warning rumbles, and Lilly stared into empty spaces with unsettling patience.

The house felt more aware with each passing hour. The quiet gathered along the walls and ceilings as if it were listening back. Christopher noticed the change immediately. Diana felt it in the pit of her stomach. Bosco tracked it with low warning rumbles, and Lilly stared into empty spaces with unsettling patience.

The house felt more aware with each passing hour. The quiet gathered along the walls and ceilings as if it were listening back. Christopher noticed the change immediately. Diana felt it in the pit of her stomach. Bosco tracked it with low warning rumbles, and Lilly stared into empty spaces with unsettling patience.

The house felt more aware with each passing hour. The quiet gathered along the walls and ceilings as if it were listening back. Christopher noticed the change immediately. Diana felt it in the pit of her stomach. Bosco tracked it with low warning rumbles, and Lilly stared into empty spaces with unsettling patience.

The house felt more aware with each passing hour. The quiet gathered along the walls and ceilings as if it were listening back. Christopher

noticed the change immediately. Diana felt it in the pit of her stomach. Bosco tracked it with low warning rumbles, and Lilly stared into empty spaces with unsettling patience.

The house felt more aware with each passing hour. The quiet gathered along the walls and ceilings as if it were listening back. Christopher noticed the change immediately. Diana felt it in the pit of her stomach. Bosco tracked it with low warning rumbles, and Lilly stared into empty spaces with unsettling patience.

It happened just after dusk.

Christopher was measuring the upper landing when the world seemed to… skip.

One moment he was marking the wall.

The next he was standing in the kitchen.

Forty-two minutes gone.

His tools had moved.

The hidden passage door stood open again.

And the thermal scanner—left upstairs—now rested on the hallway floor beside a fresh set of prints.

Diana's voice came tight over the phone. "Christopher… how did it get there?"

He stared at the device for a long time before answering.

"…I didn't move it."

The house felt more aware with each passing hour. The quiet gathered along the walls and ceilings as if it were listening back. Christopher noticed the change immediately. Diana felt it in the pit of her stomach. Bosco tracked it with low warning rumbles, and Lilly stared into empty spaces with unsettling patience.

The house felt more aware with each passing hour. The quiet gathered along the walls and ceilings as if it were listening back. Christopher noticed the change immediately. Diana felt it in the pit of her stomach. Bosco tracked it with low warning rumbles, and Lilly stared into empty spaces with unsettling patience.

The house felt more aware with each passing hour. The quiet gathered along the walls and ceilings as if it were listening back. Christopher noticed the change immediately. Diana felt it in the pit of her stomach. Bosco tracked it with low warning rumbles, and Lilly stared into empty spaces with unsettling patience.

The house felt more aware with each passing hour. The quiet gathered along the walls and ceilings as if it were listening back. Christopher noticed the change immediately. Diana felt it in the pit of her stomach. Bosco tracked it with low warning rumbles, and Lilly stared into empty spaces with unsettling patience.

The house felt more aware with each passing hour. The quiet gathered along the walls and ceilings as if it were listening back. Christopher noticed the change immediately. Diana felt it in the pit of her stomach. Bosco tracked it with low warning rumbles, and Lilly stared into empty spaces with unsettling patience.

The house felt more aware with each passing

hour. The quiet gathered along the walls and ceilings as if it were listening back. Christopher noticed the change immediately. Diana felt it in the pit of her stomach. Bosco tracked it with low warning rumbles, and Lilly stared into empty spaces with unsettling patience.

The house felt more aware with each passing hour. The quiet gathered along the walls and ceilings as if it were listening back. Christopher noticed the change immediately. Diana felt it in the pit of her stomach. Bosco tracked it with low warning rumbles, and Lilly stared into empty spaces with unsettling patience.

The house felt more aware with each passing hour. The quiet gathered along the walls and ceilings as if it were listening back. Christopher noticed the change immediately. Diana felt it in the pit of her stomach. Bosco tracked it with low warning rumbles, and Lilly stared into empty spaces with unsettling patience.

The house felt more aware with each passing hour. The quiet gathered along the walls and ceilings as if it were listening back. Christopher noticed the change immediately. Diana felt it in

the pit of her stomach. Bosco tracked it with low warning rumbles, and Lilly stared into empty spaces with unsettling patience.

The house felt more aware with each passing hour. The quiet gathered along the walls and ceilings as if it were listening back. Christopher noticed the change immediately. Diana felt it in the pit of her stomach. Bosco tracked it with low warning rumbles, and Lilly stared into empty spaces with unsettling patience.

The house felt more aware with each passing hour. The quiet gathered along the walls and ceilings as if it were listening back. Christopher noticed the change immediately. Diana felt it in the pit of her stomach. Bosco tracked it with low warning rumbles, and Lilly stared into empty spaces with unsettling patience.

The house felt more aware with each passing hour. The quiet gathered along the walls and ceilings as if it were listening back. Christopher noticed the change immediately. Diana felt it in the pit of her stomach. Bosco tracked it with low warning rumbles, and Lilly stared into empty spaces with unsettling patience.

The house felt more aware with each passing hour. The quiet gathered along the walls and ceilings as if it were listening back. Christopher noticed the change immediately. Diana felt it in the pit of her stomach. Bosco tracked it with low warning rumbles, and Lilly stared into empty spaces with unsettling patience.

The house felt more aware with each passing hour. The quiet gathered along the walls and ceilings as if it were listening back. Christopher noticed the change immediately. Diana felt it in the pit of her stomach. Bosco tracked it with low warning rumbles, and Lilly stared into empty spaces with unsettling patience.

The house felt more aware with each passing hour. The quiet gathered along the walls and ceilings as if it were listening back. Christopher noticed the change immediately. Diana felt it in the pit of her stomach. Bosco tracked it with low warning rumbles, and Lilly stared into empty spaces with unsettling patience.

The house felt more aware with each passing

hour. The quiet gathered along the walls and ceilings as if it were listening back. Christopher noticed the change immediately. Diana felt it in the pit of her stomach. Bosco tracked it with low warning rumbles, and Lilly stared into empty spaces with unsettling patience.

The house felt more aware with each passing hour. The quiet gathered along the walls and ceilings as if it were listening back. Christopher noticed the change immediately. Diana felt it in the pit of her stomach. Bosco tracked it with low warning rumbles, and Lilly stared into empty spaces with unsettling patience.

The house felt more aware with each passing hour. The quiet gathered along the walls and ceilings as if it were listening back. Christopher noticed the change immediately. Diana felt it in the pit of her stomach. Bosco tracked it with low warning rumbles, and Lilly stared into empty spaces with unsettling patience.

The house felt more aware with each passing hour. The quiet gathered along the walls and ceilings as if it were listening back. Christopher noticed the change immediately. Diana felt it in

the pit of her stomach. Bosco tracked it with low warning rumbles, and Lilly stared into empty spaces with unsettling patience.

The house felt more aware with each passing hour. The quiet gathered along the walls and ceilings as if it were listening back. Christopher noticed the change immediately. Diana felt it in the pit of her stomach. Bosco tracked it with low warning rumbles, and Lilly stared into empty spaces with unsettling patience.

The House That Watches — Chapter 10: The Camera Glitch

They reviewed every second of footage that night.

At 2:11 a.m., the upstairs camera glitched.

Not static.

Not distortion.

The time stamp froze for exactly four seconds.

When it resumed, the hallway was empty.

But the dust told a different story.

A new footprint had appeared mid-floor.

Fully formed.

No approach.

No exit trail.

Christopher leaned back slowly.

Diana's breath caught.

Because Bosco had started growling again—

Before the glitch even happened.

And Lilly…

Was staring directly into the space where the print had formed.

The house felt more aware with each passing hour. The quiet gathered along the walls and ceilings as if it were listening back. Christopher noticed the change immediately. Diana felt it in the pit of her stomach. Bosco tracked it with low warning rumbles, and Lilly stared into empty spaces with unsettling patience.

The house felt more aware with each passing hour. The quiet gathered along the walls and ceilings as if it were listening back. Christopher noticed the change immediately. Diana felt it in the pit of her stomach. Bosco tracked it with low warning rumbles, and Lilly stared into empty spaces with unsettling patience.

The house felt more aware with each passing hour. The quiet gathered along the walls and ceilings as if it were listening back. Christopher noticed the change immediately. Diana felt it in the pit of her stomach. Bosco tracked it with low warning rumbles, and Lilly stared into empty spaces with unsettling patience.

The house felt more aware with each passing hour. The quiet gathered along the walls and ceilings as if it were listening back. Christopher

noticed the change immediately. Diana felt it in the pit of her stomach. Bosco tracked it with low warning rumbles, and Lilly stared into empty spaces with unsettling patience.

The house felt more aware with each passing hour. The quiet gathered along the walls and ceilings as if it were listening back. Christopher noticed the change immediately. Diana felt it in the pit of her stomach. Bosco tracked it with low warning rumbles, and Lilly stared into empty spaces with unsettling patience.

The house felt more aware with each passing hour. The quiet gathered along the walls and ceilings as if it were listening back. Christopher noticed the change immediately. Diana felt it in the pit of her stomach. Bosco tracked it with low warning rumbles, and Lilly stared into empty spaces with unsettling patience.

The house felt more aware with each passing hour. The quiet gathered along the walls and ceilings as if it were listening back. Christopher noticed the change immediately. Diana felt it in the pit of her stomach. Bosco tracked it with low warning rumbles, and Lilly stared into empty

spaces with unsettling patience.

The house felt more aware with each passing hour. The quiet gathered along the walls and ceilings as if it were listening back. Christopher noticed the change immediately. Diana felt it in the pit of her stomach. Bosco tracked it with low warning rumbles, and Lilly stared into empty spaces with unsettling patience.

The house felt more aware with each passing hour. The quiet gathered along the walls and ceilings as if it were listening back. Christopher noticed the change immediately. Diana felt it in the pit of her stomach. Bosco tracked it with low warning rumbles, and Lilly stared into empty spaces with unsettling patience.

The house felt more aware with each passing hour. The quiet gathered along the walls and ceilings as if it were listening back. Christopher noticed the change immediately. Diana felt it in the pit of her stomach. Bosco tracked it with low warning rumbles, and Lilly stared into empty spaces with unsettling patience.

The house felt more aware with each passing hour. The quiet gathered along the walls and ceilings as if it were listening back. Christopher noticed the change immediately. Diana felt it in the pit of her stomach. Bosco tracked it with low warning rumbles, and Lilly stared into empty spaces with unsettling patience.

The house felt more aware with each passing hour. The quiet gathered along the walls and ceilings as if it were listening back. Christopher noticed the change immediately. Diana felt it in the pit of her stomach. Bosco tracked it with low warning rumbles, and Lilly stared into empty spaces with unsettling patience.

The house felt more aware with each passing hour. The quiet gathered along the walls and ceilings as if it were listening back. Christopher noticed the change immediately. Diana felt it in the pit of her stomach. Bosco tracked it with low warning rumbles, and Lilly stared into empty spaces with unsettling patience.

The house felt more aware with each passing hour. The quiet gathered along the walls and ceilings as if it were listening back. Christopher

noticed the change immediately. Diana felt it in the pit of her stomach. Bosco tracked it with low warning rumbles, and Lilly stared into empty spaces with unsettling patience.

The house felt more aware with each passing hour. The quiet gathered along the walls and ceilings as if it were listening back. Christopher noticed the change immediately. Diana felt it in the pit of her stomach. Bosco tracked it with low warning rumbles, and Lilly stared into empty spaces with unsettling patience.

The house felt more aware with each passing hour. The quiet gathered along the walls and ceilings as if it were listening back. Christopher noticed the change immediately. Diana felt it in the pit of her stomach. Bosco tracked it with low warning rumbles, and Lilly stared into empty spaces with unsettling patience.

The house felt more aware with each passing hour. The quiet gathered along the walls and ceilings as if it were listening back. Christopher noticed the change immediately. Diana felt it in the pit of her stomach. Bosco tracked it with low warning rumbles, and Lilly stared into empty

spaces with unsettling patience.

The house felt more aware with each passing hour. The quiet gathered along the walls and ceilings as if it were listening back. Christopher noticed the change immediately. Diana felt it in the pit of her stomach. Bosco tracked it with low warning rumbles, and Lilly stared into empty spaces with unsettling patience.

The house felt more aware with each passing hour. The quiet gathered along the walls and ceilings as if it were listening back. Christopher noticed the change immediately. Diana felt it in the pit of her stomach. Bosco tracked it with low warning rumbles, and Lilly stared into empty spaces with unsettling patience.

The house felt more aware with each passing hour. The quiet gathered along the walls and ceilings as if it were listening back. Christopher noticed the change immediately. Diana felt it in the pit of her stomach. Bosco tracked it with low warning rumbles, and Lilly stared into empty spaces with unsettling patience.

The sound started just after midnight.

Not loud. Not dramatic.

A slow metallic shift somewhere inside the ventilation system that ran between the floors.

Christopher froze in the upstairs hallway, head tilted slightly, listening with the same

careful attention he used when diagnosing structural problems.

"This isn't airflow," he said quietly.

Diana stood near the stairwell, arms tight across her chest. "Then what is it?"

Christopher didn't answer.

Because the sound moved.

Not randomly through the ductwork.

But in a smooth, deliberate path…

Heading toward the second-floor landing.

Bosco's growl rose instantly.

Lilly turned her head in perfect sync with the movement overhead.

The house no longer felt passive. The quiet seemed to gather with intent, pressing into the corners and lingering in the ceiling spaces as if something inside the structure was slowly becoming aware of them. Christopher noticed the shift immediately. Diana felt it in the pit of her stomach. Bosco tracked it with low warning rumbles, and Lilly watched the empty spaces as if waiting for them to move.

The house no longer felt passive. The quiet seemed to gather with intent, pressing into the corners and lingering in the ceiling spaces as if something inside the structure was slowly becoming aware of them. Christopher noticed the shift immediately. Diana felt it in the pit of her stomach. Bosco tracked it with low warning rumbles, and Lilly watched the empty spaces as if waiting for them to move.

The house no longer felt passive. The quiet seemed to gather with intent, pressing into the corners and lingering in the ceiling spaces as if something inside the structure was slowly becoming aware of them. Christopher noticed the shift immediately. Diana felt it in the pit of her stomach. Bosco tracked it with low warning rumbles, and Lilly watched the empty spaces as if waiting for them to move.

The house no longer felt passive. The quiet seemed to gather with intent, pressing into the corners and lingering in the ceiling spaces as if something inside the structure was slowly becoming aware of them. Christopher noticed the shift immediately. Diana felt it in the pit of her stomach. Bosco tracked it with low warning

rumbles, and Lilly watched the empty spaces as
if waiting for them to move.

The house no longer felt passive. The quiet
seemed to gather with intent, pressing into the
corners and lingering in the ceiling spaces as
if something inside the structure was slowly
becoming aware of them. Christopher noticed
the shift immediately. Diana felt it in the pit of
her stomach. Bosco tracked it with low warning
rumbles, and Lilly watched the empty spaces as
if waiting for them to move.

The house no longer felt passive. The quiet
seemed to gather with intent, pressing into the
corners and lingering in the ceiling spaces as
if something inside the structure was slowly
becoming aware of them. Christopher noticed
the shift immediately. Diana felt it in the pit of
her stomach. Bosco tracked it with low warning
rumbles, and Lilly watched the empty spaces as
if waiting for them to move.

The house no longer felt passive. The quiet
seemed to gather with intent, pressing into the
corners and lingering in the ceiling spaces as
if something inside the structure was slowly

becoming aware of them. Christopher noticed the shift immediately. Diana felt it in the pit of her stomach. Bosco tracked it with low warning rumbles, and Lilly watched the empty spaces as if waiting for them to move.

The house no longer felt passive. The quiet seemed to gather with intent, pressing into the corners and lingering in the ceiling spaces as if something inside the structure was slowly becoming aware of them. Christopher noticed the shift immediately. Diana felt it in the pit of her stomach. Bosco tracked it with low warning rumbles, and Lilly watched the empty spaces as if waiting for them to move.

The house no longer felt passive. The quiet seemed to gather with intent, pressing into the corners and lingering in the ceiling spaces as if something inside the structure was slowly becoming aware of them. Christopher noticed the shift immediately. Diana felt it in the pit of her stomach. Bosco tracked it with low warning rumbles, and Lilly watched the empty spaces as if waiting for them to move.

The house no longer felt passive. The quiet

seemed to gather with intent, pressing into the corners and lingering in the ceiling spaces as if something inside the structure was slowly becoming aware of them. Christopher noticed the shift immediately. Diana felt it in the pit of her stomach. Bosco tracked it with low warning rumbles, and Lilly watched the empty spaces as if waiting for them to move.

The house no longer felt passive. The quiet seemed to gather with intent, pressing into the corners and lingering in the ceiling spaces as if something inside the structure was slowly becoming aware of them. Christopher noticed the shift immediately. Diana felt it in the pit of her stomach. Bosco tracked it with low warning rumbles, and Lilly watched the empty spaces as if waiting for them to move.

The house no longer felt passive. The quiet seemed to gather with intent, pressing into the corners and lingering in the ceiling spaces as if something inside the structure was slowly becoming aware of them. Christopher noticed the shift immediately. Diana felt it in the pit of her stomach. Bosco tracked it with low warning rumbles, and Lilly watched the empty spaces as if waiting for them to move.

The house no longer felt passive. The quiet seemed to gather with intent, pressing into the corners and lingering in the ceiling spaces as if something inside the structure was slowly becoming aware of them. Christopher noticed the shift immediately. Diana felt it in the pit of her stomach. Bosco tracked it with low warning rumbles, and Lilly watched the empty spaces as if waiting for them to move.

The house no longer felt passive. The quiet seemed to gather with intent, pressing into the corners and lingering in the ceiling spaces as if something inside the structure was slowly becoming aware of them. Christopher noticed the shift immediately. Diana felt it in the pit of her stomach. Bosco tracked it with low warning rumbles, and Lilly watched the empty spaces as if waiting for them to move.

The house no longer felt passive. The quiet seemed to gather with intent, pressing into the corners and lingering in the ceiling spaces as if something inside the structure was slowly becoming aware of them. Christopher noticed the shift immediately. Diana felt it in the pit of her stomach. Bosco tracked it with low warning

rumbles, and Lilly watched the empty spaces as if waiting for them to move.

Lenny didn't want to talk about 1965.

That alone told Diana everything she needed to know.

They sat in the back booth at The Blue Jay, the low hum of conversation around them

feeling strangely far away.

"The Keller case was never clean," Lenny admitted finally. "Guy didn't just vanish.

He was working on the house the week before he disappeared."

Christopher leaned forward slightly. "Working where?"

Lenny's eyes flicked toward them.

"…inside the walls."

Silence settled heavily between them.

Because that detail had never been in the official reports.

The house no longer felt passive. The quiet seemed to gather with intent, pressing into the corners and lingering in the ceiling spaces as if something inside the structure was slowly becoming aware of them. Christopher noticed the shift immediately. Diana felt it in the pit of her stomach. Bosco tracked it with low warning rumbles, and Lilly watched the empty spaces as if waiting for them to move.

The house no longer felt passive. The quiet seemed to gather with intent, pressing into the corners and lingering in the ceiling spaces as if something inside the structure was slowly becoming aware of them. Christopher noticed the shift immediately. Diana felt it in the pit of her stomach. Bosco tracked it with low warning rumbles, and Lilly watched the empty spaces as

if waiting for them to move.

The house no longer felt passive. The quiet seemed to gather with intent, pressing into the corners and lingering in the ceiling spaces as if something inside the structure was slowly becoming aware of them. Christopher noticed the shift immediately. Diana felt it in the pit of her stomach. Bosco tracked it with low warning rumbles, and Lilly watched the empty spaces as if waiting for them to move.

The house no longer felt passive. The quiet seemed to gather with intent, pressing into the corners and lingering in the ceiling spaces as if something inside the structure was slowly becoming aware of them. Christopher noticed the shift immediately. Diana felt it in the pit of her stomach. Bosco tracked it with low warning rumbles, and Lilly watched the empty spaces as if waiting for them to move.

The house no longer felt passive. The quiet seemed to gather with intent, pressing into the corners and lingering in the ceiling spaces as if something inside the structure was slowly becoming aware of them. Christopher noticed

the shift immediately. Diana felt it in the pit of her stomach. Bosco tracked it with low warning rumbles, and Lilly watched the empty spaces as if waiting for them to move.

The house no longer felt passive. The quiet seemed to gather with intent, pressing into the corners and lingering in the ceiling spaces as if something inside the structure was slowly becoming aware of them. Christopher noticed the shift immediately. Diana felt it in the pit of her stomach. Bosco tracked it with low warning rumbles, and Lilly watched the empty spaces as if waiting for them to move.

The house no longer felt passive. The quiet seemed to gather with intent, pressing into the corners and lingering in the ceiling spaces as if something inside the structure was slowly becoming aware of them. Christopher noticed the shift immediately. Diana felt it in the pit of her stomach. Bosco tracked it with low warning rumbles, and Lilly watched the empty spaces as if waiting for them to move.

The house no longer felt passive. The quiet seemed to gather with intent, pressing into the corners and lingering in the ceiling spaces as if something inside the structure was slowly becoming aware of them. Christopher noticed the shift immediately. Diana felt it in the pit of her stomach. Bosco tracked it with low warning rumbles, and Lilly watched the empty spaces as if waiting for them to move.

The house no longer felt passive. The quiet seemed to gather with intent, pressing into the corners and lingering in the ceiling spaces as if something inside the structure was slowly becoming aware of them. Christopher noticed the shift immediately. Diana felt it in the pit of her stomach. Bosco tracked it with low warning rumbles, and Lilly watched the empty spaces as if waiting for them to move.

The house no longer felt passive. The quiet seemed to gather with intent, pressing into the corners and lingering in the ceiling spaces as if something inside the structure was slowly becoming aware of them. Christopher noticed the shift immediately. Diana felt it in the pit of her stomach. Bosco tracked it with low warning rumbles, and Lilly watched the empty spaces as if waiting for them to move.

The house no longer felt passive. The quiet seemed to gather with intent, pressing into the corners and lingering in the ceiling spaces as if something inside the structure was slowly becoming aware of them. Christopher noticed the shift immediately. Diana felt it in the pit of her stomach. Bosco tracked it with low warning rumbles, and Lilly watched the empty spaces as if waiting for them to move.

The house no longer felt passive. The quiet seemed to gather with intent, pressing into the corners and lingering in the ceiling spaces as if something inside the structure was slowly becoming aware of them. Christopher noticed the shift immediately. Diana felt it in the pit of her stomach. Bosco tracked it with low warning rumbles, and Lilly watched the empty spaces as if waiting for them to move.

The house no longer felt passive. The quiet seemed to gather with intent, pressing into the corners and lingering in the ceiling spaces as if something inside the structure was slowly becoming aware of them. Christopher noticed the shift immediately. Diana felt it in the pit of her stomach. Bosco tracked it with low warning rumbles, and Lilly watched the empty spaces as

if waiting for them to move.

The house no longer felt passive. The quiet seemed to gather with intent, pressing into the corners and lingering in the ceiling spaces as if something inside the structure was slowly becoming aware of them. Christopher noticed the shift immediately. Diana felt it in the pit of her stomach. Bosco tracked it with low warning rumbles, and Lilly watched the empty spaces as if waiting for them to move.

The house no longer felt passive. The quiet seemed to gather with intent, pressing into the corners and lingering in the ceiling spaces as if something inside the structure was slowly becoming aware of them. Christopher noticed the shift immediately. Diana felt it in the pit of her stomach. Bosco tracked it with low warning rumbles, and Lilly watched the empty spaces as if waiting for them to move.

By the end of the week, Bosco refused the blue
house entirely.

Not hesitation.

Not caution.

Refusal.

He planted his paws at the front threshold and
would not move forward no matter how

gently Diana coaxed him.

Christopher crouched beside the dog, studying
his posture.

"He's not scared," Christopher said slowly.

Diana looked down. "Then what is it?"

Christopher's jaw tightened slightly.

"…he's warning us."

Inside the house, something shifted faintly behind the walls.

And Bosco's growl deepened into something far more serious.

The house no longer felt passive. The quiet seemed to gather with intent, pressing into the corners and lingering in the ceiling spaces as if something inside the structure was slowly becoming aware of them. Christopher noticed the shift immediately. Diana felt it in the pit of her stomach. Bosco tracked it with low warning rumbles, and Lilly watched the empty spaces as if waiting for them to move.

The house no longer felt passive. The quiet seemed to gather with intent, pressing into the corners and lingering in the ceiling spaces as if something inside the structure was slowly becoming aware of them. Christopher noticed the shift immediately. Diana felt it in the pit of her stomach. Bosco tracked it with low warning rumbles, and Lilly watched the empty spaces as if waiting for them to move.

The house no longer felt passive. The quiet seemed to gather with intent, pressing into the corners and lingering in the ceiling spaces as if something inside the structure was slowly becoming aware of them. Christopher noticed the shift immediately. Diana felt it in the pit of her stomach. Bosco tracked it with low warning rumbles, and Lilly watched the empty spaces as if waiting for them to move.

The house no longer felt passive. The quiet seemed to gather with intent, pressing into the corners and lingering in the ceiling spaces as if something inside the structure was slowly becoming aware of them. Christopher noticed the shift immediately. Diana felt it in the pit of her stomach. Bosco tracked it with low warning rumbles, and Lilly watched the empty spaces as

if waiting for them to move.

The house no longer felt passive. The quiet seemed to gather with intent, pressing into the corners and lingering in the ceiling spaces as if something inside the structure was slowly becoming aware of them. Christopher noticed the shift immediately. Diana felt it in the pit of her stomach. Bosco tracked it with low warning rumbles, and Lilly watched the empty spaces as if waiting for them to move.

The house no longer felt passive. The quiet seemed to gather with intent, pressing into the corners and lingering in the ceiling spaces as if something inside the structure was slowly becoming aware of them. Christopher noticed the shift immediately. Diana felt it in the pit of her stomach. Bosco tracked it with low warning rumbles, and Lilly watched the empty spaces as if waiting for them to move.

The house no longer felt passive. The quiet seemed to gather with intent, pressing into the corners and lingering in the ceiling spaces as if something inside the structure was slowly becoming aware of them. Christopher noticed

the shift immediately. Diana felt it in the pit of her stomach. Bosco tracked it with low warning rumbles, and Lilly watched the empty spaces as if waiting for them to move.

The house no longer felt passive. The quiet seemed to gather with intent, pressing into the corners and lingering in the ceiling spaces as if something inside the structure was slowly becoming aware of them. Christopher noticed the shift immediately. Diana felt it in the pit of her stomach. Bosco tracked it with low warning rumbles, and Lilly watched the empty spaces as if waiting for them to move.

The house no longer felt passive. The quiet seemed to gather with intent, pressing into the corners and lingering in the ceiling spaces as if something inside the structure was slowly becoming aware of them. Christopher noticed the shift immediately. Diana felt it in the pit of her stomach. Bosco tracked it with low warning rumbles, and Lilly watched the empty spaces as if waiting for them to move.

The house no longer felt passive. The quiet seemed to gather with intent, pressing into the corners and lingering in the ceiling spaces as if something inside the structure was slowly becoming aware of them. Christopher noticed the shift immediately. Diana felt it in the pit of her stomach. Bosco tracked it with low warning rumbles, and Lilly watched the empty spaces as if waiting for them to move.

The house no longer felt passive. The quiet seemed to gather with intent, pressing into the corners and lingering in the ceiling spaces as if something inside the structure was slowly becoming aware of them. Christopher noticed the shift immediately. Diana felt it in the pit of her stomach. Bosco tracked it with low warning rumbles, and Lilly watched the empty spaces as if waiting for them to move.

The house no longer felt passive. The quiet seemed to gather with intent, pressing into the corners and lingering in the ceiling spaces as if something inside the structure was slowly becoming aware of them. Christopher noticed the shift immediately. Diana felt it in the pit of her stomach. Bosco tracked it with low warning rumbles, and Lilly watched the empty spaces as if waiting for them to move.

The house no longer felt passive. The quiet seemed to gather with intent, pressing into the corners and lingering in the ceiling spaces as if something inside the structure was slowly becoming aware of them. Christopher noticed the shift immediately. Diana felt it in the pit of her stomach. Bosco tracked it with low warning rumbles, and Lilly watched the empty spaces as if waiting for them to move.

The house no longer felt passive. The quiet seemed to gather with intent, pressing into the corners and lingering in the ceiling spaces as if something inside the structure was slowly becoming aware of them. Christopher noticed the shift immediately. Diana felt it in the pit of her stomach. Bosco tracked it with low warning rumbles, and Lilly watched the empty spaces as if waiting for them to move.

The house no longer felt passive. The quiet seemed to gather with intent, pressing into the corners and lingering in the ceiling spaces as if something inside the structure was slowly becoming aware of them. Christopher noticed the shift immediately. Diana felt it in the pit of her stomach. Bosco tracked it with low warning rumbles, and Lilly watched the empty spaces as

if waiting for them to move.

The House That Watches — Chapter 14: Lilly's Fixation

If Bosco was the alarm, Lilly was the observer.

For nearly twenty minutes she sat motionless in the upstairs hallway, eyes fixed on a

single section of wall just above the baseboard.

Christopher followed her gaze.

At first, he saw nothing.

Then the thermal scanner flickered.

A narrow cold ribbon traced slowly upward inside the wall cavity.

Moving.

Steady.

Intentional.

Diana's voice dropped to a whisper.

"…it knows where we are now."

The house no longer felt passive. The quiet seemed to gather with intent, pressing into the corners and lingering in the ceiling spaces as if something inside the structure was slowly becoming aware of them. Christopher noticed the shift immediately. Diana felt it in the pit of her stomach. Bosco tracked it with low warning rumbles, and Lilly watched the empty spaces as if waiting for them to move.

The house no longer felt passive. The quiet seemed to gather with intent, pressing into the corners and lingering in the ceiling spaces as if something inside the structure was slowly becoming aware of them. Christopher noticed the shift immediately. Diana felt it in the pit of her stomach. Bosco tracked it with low warning rumbles, and Lilly watched the empty spaces as if waiting for them to move.

The house no longer felt passive. The quiet seemed to gather with intent, pressing into the corners and lingering in the ceiling spaces as if something inside the structure was slowly becoming aware of them. Christopher noticed the shift immediately. Diana felt it in the pit of her stomach. Bosco tracked it with low warning rumbles, and Lilly watched the empty spaces as if waiting for them to move.

The house no longer felt passive. The quiet seemed to gather with intent, pressing into the corners and lingering in the ceiling spaces as if something inside the structure was slowly becoming aware of them. Christopher noticed the shift immediately. Diana felt it in the pit of her stomach. Bosco tracked it with low warning rumbles, and Lilly watched the empty spaces as if waiting for them to move.

The house no longer felt passive. The quiet seemed to gather with intent, pressing into the corners and lingering in the ceiling spaces as if something inside the structure was slowly becoming aware of them. Christopher noticed the shift immediately. Diana felt it in the pit of her stomach. Bosco tracked it with low warning rumbles, and Lilly watched the empty spaces as if waiting for them to move.

The house no longer felt passive. The quiet seemed to gather with intent, pressing into the corners and lingering in the ceiling spaces as if something inside the structure was slowly becoming aware of them. Christopher noticed the shift immediately. Diana felt it in the pit of her stomach. Bosco tracked it with low warning rumbles, and Lilly watched the empty spaces as if waiting for them to move.

The house no longer felt passive. The quiet seemed to gather with intent, pressing into the corners and lingering in the ceiling spaces as if something inside the structure was slowly becoming aware of them. Christopher noticed the shift immediately. Diana felt it in the pit of her stomach. Bosco tracked it with low warning rumbles, and Lilly watched the empty spaces as if waiting for them to move.

The house no longer felt passive. The quiet seemed to gather with intent, pressing into the corners and lingering in the ceiling spaces as if something inside the structure was slowly becoming aware of them. Christopher noticed the shift immediately. Diana felt it in the pit of her stomach. Bosco tracked it with low warning rumbles, and Lilly watched the empty spaces as if waiting for them to move.

The house no longer felt passive. The quiet seemed to gather with intent, pressing into the corners and lingering in the ceiling spaces as if something inside the structure was slowly becoming aware of them. Christopher noticed the shift immediately. Diana felt it in the pit of her stomach. Bosco tracked it with low warning rumbles, and Lilly watched the empty spaces as if waiting for them to move.

The house no longer felt passive. The quiet seemed to gather with intent, pressing into the corners and lingering in the ceiling spaces as if something inside the structure was slowly becoming aware of them. Christopher noticed the shift immediately. Diana felt it in the pit of her stomach. Bosco tracked it with low warning rumbles, and Lilly watched the empty spaces as

if waiting for them to move.

The house no longer felt passive. The quiet seemed to gather with intent, pressing into the corners and lingering in the ceiling spaces as if something inside the structure was slowly becoming aware of them. Christopher noticed the shift immediately. Diana felt it in the pit of her stomach. Bosco tracked it with low warning rumbles, and Lilly watched the empty spaces as if waiting for them to move.

The house no longer felt passive. The quiet seemed to gather with intent, pressing into the corners and lingering in the ceiling spaces as if something inside the structure was slowly becoming aware of them. Christopher noticed the shift immediately. Diana felt it in the pit of her stomach. Bosco tracked it with low warning rumbles, and Lilly watched the empty spaces as if waiting for them to move.

The house no longer felt passive. The quiet seemed to gather with intent, pressing into the corners and lingering in the ceiling spaces as if something inside the structure was slowly becoming aware of them. Christopher noticed

the shift immediately. Diana felt it in the pit of her stomach. Bosco tracked it with low warning rumbles, and Lilly watched the empty spaces as if waiting for them to move.

The house no longer felt passive. The quiet seemed to gather with intent, pressing into the corners and lingering in the ceiling spaces as if something inside the structure was slowly becoming aware of them. Christopher noticed the shift immediately. Diana felt it in the pit of her stomach. Bosco tracked it with low warning rumbles, and Lilly watched the empty spaces as if waiting for them to move.

The house no longer felt passive. The quiet seemed to gather with intent, pressing into the corners and lingering in the ceiling spaces as if something inside the structure was slowly becoming aware of them. Christopher noticed the shift immediately. Diana felt it in the pit of her stomach. Bosco tracked it with low warning rumbles, and Lilly watched the empty spaces as if waiting for them to move.

The House That Watches — Chapter 15: The Narrow Space

Christopher finally opened the upper seam.

The cut was careful, precise — the work of a man who still trusted physical answers.

Behind the drywall…

Was space.

Too narrow for comfort.

Too smooth to be accidental.

And running the length of the second-floor wall like a hidden corridor no blueprint

had ever recorded.

Christopher shone the flashlight deeper inside.

The beam caught dust.

Old wiring.

And something else.

Fresh disturbance marks.

Like something had passed through only minutes earlier.

The house no longer felt passive. The quiet seemed to gather with intent, pressing into the corners and lingering in the ceiling spaces as if something inside the structure was slowly becoming aware of them. Christopher noticed the shift immediately. Diana felt it in the pit of her stomach. Bosco tracked it with low warning rumbles, and Lilly watched the empty spaces as if waiting for them to move.

The house no longer felt passive. The quiet seemed to gather with intent, pressing into the corners and lingering in the ceiling spaces as if something inside the structure was slowly becoming aware of them. Christopher noticed the shift immediately. Diana felt it in the pit of her stomach. Bosco tracked it with low warning rumbles, and Lilly watched the empty spaces as if waiting for them to move.

The house no longer felt passive. The quiet seemed to gather with intent, pressing into the corners and lingering in the ceiling spaces as if something inside the structure was slowly becoming aware of them. Christopher noticed the shift immediately. Diana felt it in the pit of her stomach. Bosco tracked it with low warning rumbles, and Lilly watched the empty spaces as if waiting for them to move.

The house no longer felt passive. The quiet seemed to gather with intent, pressing into the corners and lingering in the ceiling spaces as if something inside the structure was slowly becoming aware of them. Christopher noticed the shift immediately. Diana felt it in the pit of her stomach. Bosco tracked it with low warning

rumbles, and Lilly watched the empty spaces as if waiting for them to move.

The house no longer felt passive. The quiet seemed to gather with intent, pressing into the corners and lingering in the ceiling spaces as if something inside the structure was slowly becoming aware of them. Christopher noticed the shift immediately. Diana felt it in the pit of her stomach. Bosco tracked it with low warning rumbles, and Lilly watched the empty spaces as if waiting for them to move.

The house no longer felt passive. The quiet seemed to gather with intent, pressing into the corners and lingering in the ceiling spaces as if something inside the structure was slowly becoming aware of them. Christopher noticed the shift immediately. Diana felt it in the pit of her stomach. Bosco tracked it with low warning rumbles, and Lilly watched the empty spaces as if waiting for them to move.

The house no longer felt passive. The quiet seemed to gather with intent, pressing into the corners and lingering in the ceiling spaces as if something inside the structure was slowly becoming aware of them. Christopher noticed the shift immediately. Diana felt it in the pit of her stomach. Bosco tracked it with low warning rumbles, and Lilly watched the empty spaces as if waiting for them to move.

The house no longer felt passive. The quiet seemed to gather with intent, pressing into the corners and lingering in the ceiling spaces as if something inside the structure was slowly becoming aware of them. Christopher noticed the shift immediately. Diana felt it in the pit of her stomach. Bosco tracked it with low warning rumbles, and Lilly watched the empty spaces as if waiting for them to move.

The house no longer felt passive. The quiet seemed to gather with intent, pressing into the corners and lingering in the ceiling spaces as if something inside the structure was slowly becoming aware of them. Christopher noticed the shift immediately. Diana felt it in the pit of her stomach. Bosco tracked it with low warning rumbles, and Lilly watched the empty spaces as if waiting for them to move.

The house no longer felt passive. The quiet

seemed to gather with intent, pressing into the corners and lingering in the ceiling spaces as if something inside the structure was slowly becoming aware of them. Christopher noticed the shift immediately. Diana felt it in the pit of her stomach. Bosco tracked it with low warning rumbles, and Lilly watched the empty spaces as if waiting for them to move.

The house no longer felt passive. The quiet seemed to gather with intent, pressing into the corners and lingering in the ceiling spaces as if something inside the structure was slowly becoming aware of them. Christopher noticed the shift immediately. Diana felt it in the pit of her stomach. Bosco tracked it with low warning rumbles, and Lilly watched the empty spaces as if waiting for them to move.

The house no longer felt passive. The quiet seemed to gather with intent, pressing into the corners and lingering in the ceiling spaces as if something inside the structure was slowly becoming aware of them. Christopher noticed the shift immediately. Diana felt it in the pit of her stomach. Bosco tracked it with low warning rumbles, and Lilly watched the empty spaces as if waiting for them to move.

The house no longer felt passive. The quiet seemed to gather with intent, pressing into the corners and lingering in the ceiling spaces as if something inside the structure was slowly becoming aware of them. Christopher noticed the shift immediately. Diana felt it in the pit of her stomach. Bosco tracked it with low warning rumbles, and Lilly watched the empty spaces as if waiting for them to move.

The house no longer felt passive. The quiet seemed to gather with intent, pressing into the corners and lingering in the ceiling spaces as if something inside the structure was slowly becoming aware of them. Christopher noticed the shift immediately. Diana felt it in the pit of her stomach. Bosco tracked it with low warning rumbles, and Lilly watched the empty spaces as if waiting for them to move.

The house no longer felt passive. The quiet seemed to gather with intent, pressing into the corners and lingering in the ceiling spaces as if something inside the structure was slowly becoming aware of them. Christopher noticed the shift immediately. Diana felt it in the pit of her stomach. Bosco tracked it with low warning

rumbles, and Lilly watched the empty spaces as if waiting for them to move.

The first print appeared on the front walk just after dawn.

Diana saw it when she stepped outside with Bosco, coffee still warm in her hand.

One bare footprint marked the thin layer of dust near the edge of the concrete.

Facing the house.

Her pulse jumped instantly.

Christopher was there within minutes, crouching low, studying the impression with

tight, professional focus.

"It's the same size," he said quietly.

Bosco's growl started low and stayed there.

Because whatever had been inside the walls…

Was no longer staying there.

The house felt increasingly aware of their presence. The quiet pooled in the corners and stretched through the ceiling cavities as if something inside the structure were tracking their movements. Christopher noticed the pattern immediately. Diana felt it like pressure behind her ribs. Bosco followed it with low warning rumbles, and Lilly watched the empty spaces with unnerving patience.

The house felt increasingly aware of their presence. The quiet pooled in the corners and stretched through the ceiling cavities as if something inside the structure were tracking their movements. Christopher noticed the pattern immediately. Diana felt it like pressure behind her ribs. Bosco followed it with low warning rumbles, and Lilly watched the empty spaces with unnerving patience.

The house felt increasingly aware of their presence. The quiet pooled in the corners and stretched through the ceiling cavities as if something inside the structure were tracking their movements. Christopher noticed the pattern immediately. Diana felt it like pressure behind her ribs. Bosco followed it with low warning rumbles, and Lilly watched the empty spaces with unnerving patience.

The house felt increasingly aware of their presence. The quiet pooled in the corners and stretched through the ceiling cavities as if something inside the structure were tracking their movements. Christopher noticed the pattern immediately. Diana felt it like pressure behind her ribs. Bosco followed it with low warning rumbles, and Lilly watched the empty spaces with unnerving patience.

The house felt increasingly aware of their presence. The quiet pooled in the corners and stretched through the ceiling cavities as if something inside the structure were tracking their movements. Christopher noticed the pattern immediately. Diana felt it like pressure behind her ribs. Bosco followed it with low warning

rumbles, and Lilly watched the empty spaces with unnerving patience.

The house felt increasingly aware of their presence. The quiet pooled in the corners and stretched through the ceiling cavities as if something inside the structure were tracking their movements. Christopher noticed the pattern immediately. Diana felt it like pressure behind her ribs. Bosco followed it with low warning rumbles, and Lilly watched the empty spaces with unnerving patience.

The house felt increasingly aware of their presence. The quiet pooled in the corners and stretched through the ceiling cavities as if something inside the structure were tracking their movements. Christopher noticed the pattern immediately. Diana felt it like pressure behind her ribs. Bosco followed it with low warning rumbles, and Lilly watched the empty spaces with unnerving patience.

The house felt increasingly aware of their presence. The quiet pooled in the corners and stretched through the ceiling cavities as if something inside the structure were tracking their

movements. Christopher noticed the pattern immediately. Diana felt it like pressure behind her ribs. Bosco followed it with low warning rumbles, and Lilly watched the empty spaces with unnerving patience.

The house felt increasingly aware of their presence. The quiet pooled in the corners and stretched through the ceiling cavities as if something inside the structure were tracking their movements. Christopher noticed the pattern immediately. Diana felt it like pressure behind her ribs. Bosco followed it with low warning rumbles, and Lilly watched the empty spaces with unnerving patience.

The house felt increasingly aware of their presence. The quiet pooled in the corners and stretched through the ceiling cavities as if something inside the structure were tracking their movements. Christopher noticed the pattern immediately. Diana felt it like pressure behind her ribs. Bosco followed it with low warning rumbles, and Lilly watched the empty spaces with unnerving patience.

The house felt increasingly aware of their

presence. The quiet pooled in the corners and stretched through the ceiling cavities as if something inside the structure were tracking their movements. Christopher noticed the pattern immediately. Diana felt it like pressure behind her ribs. Bosco followed it with low warning rumbles, and Lilly watched the empty spaces with unnerving patience.

The house felt increasingly aware of their presence. The quiet pooled in the corners and stretched through the ceiling cavities as if something inside the structure were tracking their movements. Christopher noticed the pattern immediately. Diana felt it like pressure behind her ribs. Bosco followed it with low warning rumbles, and Lilly watched the empty spaces with unnerving patience.

The house felt increasingly aware of their presence. The quiet pooled in the corners and stretched through the ceiling cavities as if something inside the structure were tracking their movements. Christopher noticed the pattern immediately. Diana felt it like pressure behind her ribs. Bosco followed it with low warning rumbles, and Lilly watched the empty spaces with unnerving patience.

The house felt increasingly aware of their presence. The quiet pooled in the corners and stretched through the ceiling cavities as if something inside the structure were tracking their movements. Christopher noticed the pattern immediately. Diana felt it like pressure behind her ribs. Bosco followed it with low warning rumbles, and Lilly watched the empty spaces with unnerving patience.

The house felt increasingly aware of their presence. The quiet pooled in the corners and stretched through the ceiling cavities as if something inside the structure were tracking their movements. Christopher noticed the pattern immediately. Diana felt it like pressure behind her ribs. Bosco followed it with low warning rumbles, and Lilly watched the empty spaces with unnerving patience.

The house felt increasingly aware of their presence. The quiet pooled in the corners and stretched through the ceiling cavities as if something inside the structure were tracking their movements. Christopher noticed the pattern immediately. Diana felt it like pressure behind her ribs. Bosco followed it with low warning

rumbles, and Lilly watched the empty spaces with unnerving patience.

The house felt increasingly aware of their presence. The quiet pooled in the corners and stretched through the ceiling cavities as if something inside the structure were tracking their movements. Christopher noticed the pattern immediately. Diana felt it like pressure behind her ribs. Bosco followed it with low warning rumbles, and Lilly watched the empty spaces with unnerving patience.

The house felt increasingly aware of their presence. The quiet pooled in the corners and stretched through the ceiling cavities as if something inside the structure were tracking their movements. Christopher noticed the pattern immediately. Diana felt it like pressure behind her ribs. Bosco followed it with low warning rumbles, and Lilly watched the empty spaces with unnerving patience.

Christopher installed exterior cameras that afternoon.

If the movement was spreading beyond the structure, he wanted proof.

At 1:43 a.m., the first exterior glitch appeared.

Not static.

Not interference.

The porch camera skipped forward two full seconds.

When the feed resumed, the front walkway was empty.

But the dust told a different story.

A new footprint had formed between frames.

Diana felt the cold realization settle deep.

The house wasn't just active.

It was adapting.

The house felt increasingly aware of their presence. The quiet pooled in the corners and stretched through the ceiling cavities as if something inside the structure were tracking their movements. Christopher noticed the pattern immediately. Diana felt it like pressure behind her ribs. Bosco followed it with low warning rumbles, and Lilly watched the empty spaces with unnerving patience.

The house felt increasingly aware of their presence. The quiet pooled in the corners and

stretched through the ceiling cavities as if something inside the structure were tracking their movements. Christopher noticed the pattern immediately. Diana felt it like pressure behind her ribs. Bosco followed it with low warning rumbles, and Lilly watched the empty spaces with unnerving patience.

The house felt increasingly aware of their presence. The quiet pooled in the corners and stretched through the ceiling cavities as if something inside the structure were tracking their movements. Christopher noticed the pattern immediately. Diana felt it like pressure behind her ribs. Bosco followed it with low warning rumbles, and Lilly watched the empty spaces with unnerving patience.

The house felt increasingly aware of their presence. The quiet pooled in the corners and stretched through the ceiling cavities as if something inside the structure were tracking their movements. Christopher noticed the pattern immediately. Diana felt it like pressure behind her ribs. Bosco followed it with low warning rumbles, and Lilly watched the empty spaces with unnerving patience.

The house felt increasingly aware of their presence. The quiet pooled in the corners and stretched through the ceiling cavities as if something inside the structure were tracking their movements. Christopher noticed the pattern immediately. Diana felt it like pressure behind her ribs. Bosco followed it with low warning rumbles, and Lilly watched the empty spaces with unnerving patience.

The house felt increasingly aware of their presence. The quiet pooled in the corners and stretched through the ceiling cavities as if something inside the structure were tracking their movements. Christopher noticed the pattern immediately. Diana felt it like pressure behind her ribs. Bosco followed it with low warning rumbles, and Lilly watched the empty spaces with unnerving patience.

The house felt increasingly aware of their presence. The quiet pooled in the corners and stretched through the ceiling cavities as if something inside the structure were tracking their movements. Christopher noticed the pattern immediately. Diana felt it like pressure behind her ribs. Bosco followed it with low warning rumbles, and Lilly watched the empty spaces

with unnerving patience.

The house felt increasingly aware of their presence. The quiet pooled in the corners and stretched through the ceiling cavities as if something inside the structure were tracking their movements. Christopher noticed the pattern immediately. Diana felt it like pressure behind her ribs. Bosco followed it with low warning rumbles, and Lilly watched the empty spaces with unnerving patience.

The house felt increasingly aware of their presence. The quiet pooled in the corners and stretched through the ceiling cavities as if something inside the structure were tracking their movements. Christopher noticed the pattern immediately. Diana felt it like pressure behind her ribs. Bosco followed it with low warning rumbles, and Lilly watched the empty spaces with unnerving patience.

The house felt increasingly aware of their presence. The quiet pooled in the corners and stretched through the ceiling cavities as if something inside the structure were tracking their movements. Christopher noticed the pattern

immediately. Diana felt it like pressure behind her ribs. Bosco followed it with low warning rumbles, and Lilly watched the empty spaces with unnerving patience.

The house felt increasingly aware of their presence. The quiet pooled in the corners and stretched through the ceiling cavities as if something inside the structure were tracking their movements. Christopher noticed the pattern immediately. Diana felt it like pressure behind her ribs. Bosco followed it with low warning rumbles, and Lilly watched the empty spaces with unnerving patience.

The house felt increasingly aware of their presence. The quiet pooled in the corners and stretched through the ceiling cavities as if something inside the structure were tracking their movements. Christopher noticed the pattern immediately. Diana felt it like pressure behind her ribs. Bosco followed it with low warning rumbles, and Lilly watched the empty spaces with unnerving patience.

The house felt increasingly aware of their presence. The quiet pooled in the corners and

stretched through the ceiling cavities as if something inside the structure were tracking their movements. Christopher noticed the pattern immediately. Diana felt it like pressure behind her ribs. Bosco followed it with low warning rumbles, and Lilly watched the empty spaces with unnerving patience.

The house felt increasingly aware of their presence. The quiet pooled in the corners and stretched through the ceiling cavities as if something inside the structure were tracking their movements. Christopher noticed the pattern immediately. Diana felt it like pressure behind her ribs. Bosco followed it with low warning rumbles, and Lilly watched the empty spaces with unnerving patience.

The house felt increasingly aware of their presence. The quiet pooled in the corners and stretched through the ceiling cavities as if something inside the structure were tracking their movements. Christopher noticed the pattern immediately. Diana felt it like pressure behind her ribs. Bosco followed it with low warning rumbles, and Lilly watched the empty spaces with unnerving patience.

The house felt increasingly aware of their presence. The quiet pooled in the corners and stretched through the ceiling cavities as if something inside the structure were tracking their movements. Christopher noticed the pattern immediately. Diana felt it like pressure behind her ribs. Bosco followed it with low warning rumbles, and Lilly watched the empty spaces with unnerving patience.

The house felt increasingly aware of their presence. The quiet pooled in the corners and stretched through the ceiling cavities as if something inside the structure were tracking their movements. Christopher noticed the pattern immediately. Diana felt it like pressure behind her ribs. Bosco followed it with low warning rumbles, and Lilly watched the empty spaces with unnerving patience.

The house felt increasingly aware of their presence. The quiet pooled in the corners and stretched through the ceiling cavities as if something inside the structure were tracking their movements. Christopher noticed the pattern immediately. Diana felt it like pressure behind her ribs. Bosco followed it with low warning rumbles, and Lilly watched the empty spaces

with unnerving patience.

Lenny was the one who said it first.

Too casually.

Too carefully.

"You ever notice," he said slowly, "how close the original Keller property lines ran?"

Christopher looked up sharply.

Lenny tapped the old neighborhood map once.

"The modifications didn't stop at the blue house."

Silence fell hard in the room.

Because the property lines overlapped three adjacent structures.

Including Diana's townhouse.

Bosco began barking before anyone spoke again.

The house felt increasingly aware of their presence. The quiet pooled in the corners and stretched through the ceiling cavities as if something inside the structure were tracking their movements. Christopher noticed the pattern immediately. Diana felt it like pressure behind her ribs. Bosco followed it with low warning rumbles, and Lilly watched the empty spaces with unnerving patience.

The house felt increasingly aware of their presence. The quiet pooled in the corners and stretched through the ceiling cavities as if something inside the structure were tracking their movements. Christopher noticed the pattern immediately. Diana felt it like pressure behind her ribs. Bosco followed it with low warning rumbles, and Lilly watched the empty spaces

with unnerving patience.

The house felt increasingly aware of their presence. The quiet pooled in the corners and stretched through the ceiling cavities as if something inside the structure were tracking their movements. Christopher noticed the pattern immediately. Diana felt it like pressure behind her ribs. Bosco followed it with low warning rumbles, and Lilly watched the empty spaces with unnerving patience.

The house felt increasingly aware of their presence. The quiet pooled in the corners and stretched through the ceiling cavities as if something inside the structure were tracking their movements. Christopher noticed the pattern immediately. Diana felt it like pressure behind her ribs. Bosco followed it with low warning rumbles, and Lilly watched the empty spaces with unnerving patience.

The house felt increasingly aware of their presence. The quiet pooled in the corners and stretched through the ceiling cavities as if something inside the structure were tracking their movements. Christopher noticed the pattern

immediately. Diana felt it like pressure behind her ribs. Bosco followed it with low warning rumbles, and Lilly watched the empty spaces with unnerving patience.

The house felt increasingly aware of their presence. The quiet pooled in the corners and stretched through the ceiling cavities as if something inside the structure were tracking their movements. Christopher noticed the pattern immediately. Diana felt it like pressure behind her ribs. Bosco followed it with low warning rumbles, and Lilly watched the empty spaces with unnerving patience.

The house felt increasingly aware of their presence. The quiet pooled in the corners and stretched through the ceiling cavities as if something inside the structure were tracking their movements. Christopher noticed the pattern immediately. Diana felt it like pressure behind her ribs. Bosco followed it with low warning rumbles, and Lilly watched the empty spaces with unnerving patience.

The house felt increasingly aware of their presence. The quiet pooled in the corners and

stretched through the ceiling cavities as if something inside the structure were tracking their movements. Christopher noticed the pattern immediately. Diana felt it like pressure behind her ribs. Bosco followed it with low warning rumbles, and Lilly watched the empty spaces with unnerving patience.

The house felt increasingly aware of their presence. The quiet pooled in the corners and stretched through the ceiling cavities as if something inside the structure were tracking their movements. Christopher noticed the pattern immediately. Diana felt it like pressure behind her ribs. Bosco followed it with low warning rumbles, and Lilly watched the empty spaces with unnerving patience.

The house felt increasingly aware of their presence. The quiet pooled in the corners and stretched through the ceiling cavities as if something inside the structure were tracking their movements. Christopher noticed the pattern immediately. Diana felt it like pressure behind her ribs. Bosco followed it with low warning rumbles, and Lilly watched the empty spaces with unnerving patience.

The house felt increasingly aware of their presence. The quiet pooled in the corners and stretched through the ceiling cavities as if something inside the structure were tracking their movements. Christopher noticed the pattern immediately. Diana felt it like pressure behind her ribs. Bosco followed it with low warning rumbles, and Lilly watched the empty spaces with unnerving patience.

The house felt increasingly aware of their presence. The quiet pooled in the corners and stretched through the ceiling cavities as if something inside the structure were tracking their movements. Christopher noticed the pattern immediately. Diana felt it like pressure behind her ribs. Bosco followed it with low warning rumbles, and Lilly watched the empty spaces with unnerving patience.

The house felt increasingly aware of their presence. The quiet pooled in the corners and stretched through the ceiling cavities as if something inside the structure were tracking their movements. Christopher noticed the pattern immediately. Diana felt it like pressure behind her ribs. Bosco followed it with low warning rumbles, and Lilly watched the empty spaces

with unnerving patience.

The house felt increasingly aware of their presence. The quiet pooled in the corners and stretched through the ceiling cavities as if something inside the structure were tracking their movements. Christopher noticed the pattern immediately. Diana felt it like pressure behind her ribs. Bosco followed it with low warning rumbles, and Lilly watched the empty spaces with unnerving patience.

The house felt increasingly aware of their presence. The quiet pooled in the corners and stretched through the ceiling cavities as if something inside the structure were tracking their movements. Christopher noticed the pattern immediately. Diana felt it like pressure behind her ribs. Bosco followed it with low warning rumbles, and Lilly watched the empty spaces with unnerving patience.

The house felt increasingly aware of their presence. The quiet pooled in the corners and stretched through the ceiling cavities as if something inside the structure were tracking their movements. Christopher noticed the pattern

immediately. Diana felt it like pressure behind her ribs. Bosco followed it with low warning rumbles, and Lilly watched the empty spaces with unnerving patience.

The house felt increasingly aware of their presence. The quiet pooled in the corners and stretched through the ceiling cavities as if something inside the structure were tracking their movements. Christopher noticed the pattern immediately. Diana felt it like pressure behind her ribs. Bosco followed it with low warning rumbles, and Lilly watched the empty spaces with unnerving patience.

The house felt increasingly aware of their presence. The quiet pooled in the corners and stretched through the ceiling cavities as if something inside the structure were tracking their movements. Christopher noticed the pattern immediately. Diana felt it like pressure behind her ribs. Bosco followed it with low warning rumbles, and Lilly watched the empty spaces with unnerving patience.

Thermal readings confirmed it.

Cold ribbons were beginning to appear inside Diana's townhouse walls — faint, narrow,

but unmistakably similar to the patterns inside the blue house.

Christopher ran the scanner twice.

Then a third time.

The readings didn't change.

Diana's voice dropped to a whisper.

"…it followed us."

From somewhere inside her living room wall, a soft shifting sound answered.

The house felt increasingly aware of their presence. The quiet pooled in the corners and stretched through the ceiling cavities as if something inside the structure were tracking their movements. Christopher noticed the pattern immediately. Diana felt it like pressure behind her ribs. Bosco followed it with low warning rumbles, and Lilly watched the empty spaces with unnerving patience.

The house felt increasingly aware of their presence. The quiet pooled in the corners and stretched through the ceiling cavities as if something inside the structure were tracking their movements. Christopher noticed the pattern immediately. Diana felt it like pressure behind her ribs. Bosco followed it with low warning rumbles, and Lilly watched the empty spaces with unnerving patience.

The house felt increasingly aware of their presence. The quiet pooled in the corners and stretched through the ceiling cavities as if something inside the structure were tracking their

movements. Christopher noticed the pattern immediately. Diana felt it like pressure behind her ribs. Bosco followed it with low warning rumbles, and Lilly watched the empty spaces with unnerving patience.

The house felt increasingly aware of their presence. The quiet pooled in the corners and stretched through the ceiling cavities as if something inside the structure were tracking their movements. Christopher noticed the pattern immediately. Diana felt it like pressure behind her ribs. Bosco followed it with low warning rumbles, and Lilly watched the empty spaces with unnerving patience.

The house felt increasingly aware of their presence. The quiet pooled in the corners and stretched through the ceiling cavities as if something inside the structure were tracking their movements. Christopher noticed the pattern immediately. Diana felt it like pressure behind her ribs. Bosco followed it with low warning rumbles, and Lilly watched the empty spaces with unnerving patience.

The house felt increasingly aware of their

presence. The quiet pooled in the corners and stretched through the ceiling cavities as if something inside the structure were tracking their movements. Christopher noticed the pattern immediately. Diana felt it like pressure behind her ribs. Bosco followed it with low warning rumbles, and Lilly watched the empty spaces with unnerving patience.

The house felt increasingly aware of their presence. The quiet pooled in the corners and stretched through the ceiling cavities as if something inside the structure were tracking their movements. Christopher noticed the pattern immediately. Diana felt it like pressure behind her ribs. Bosco followed it with low warning rumbles, and Lilly watched the empty spaces with unnerving patience.

The house felt increasingly aware of their presence. The quiet pooled in the corners and stretched through the ceiling cavities as if something inside the structure were tracking their movements. Christopher noticed the pattern immediately. Diana felt it like pressure behind her ribs. Bosco followed it with low warning rumbles, and Lilly watched the empty spaces with unnerving patience.

The house felt increasingly aware of their presence. The quiet pooled in the corners and stretched through the ceiling cavities as if something inside the structure were tracking their movements. Christopher noticed the pattern immediately. Diana felt it like pressure behind her ribs. Bosco followed it with low warning rumbles, and Lilly watched the empty spaces with unnerving patience.

The house felt increasingly aware of their presence. The quiet pooled in the corners and stretched through the ceiling cavities as if something inside the structure were tracking their movements. Christopher noticed the pattern immediately. Diana felt it like pressure behind her ribs. Bosco followed it with low warning rumbles, and Lilly watched the empty spaces with unnerving patience.

The house felt increasingly aware of their presence. The quiet pooled in the corners and stretched through the ceiling cavities as if something inside the structure were tracking their movements. Christopher noticed the pattern immediately. Diana felt it like pressure behind her ribs. Bosco followed it with low warning

rumbles, and Lilly watched the empty spaces with unnerving patience.

The house felt increasingly aware of their presence. The quiet pooled in the corners and stretched through the ceiling cavities as if something inside the structure were tracking their movements. Christopher noticed the pattern immediately. Diana felt it like pressure behind her ribs. Bosco followed it with low warning rumbles, and Lilly watched the empty spaces with unnerving patience.

The house felt increasingly aware of their presence. The quiet pooled in the corners and stretched through the ceiling cavities as if something inside the structure were tracking their movements. Christopher noticed the pattern immediately. Diana felt it like pressure behind her ribs. Bosco followed it with low warning rumbles, and Lilly watched the empty spaces with unnerving patience.

The house felt increasingly aware of their presence. The quiet pooled in the corners and stretched through the ceiling cavities as if something inside the structure were tracking their

movements. Christopher noticed the pattern immediately. Diana felt it like pressure behind her ribs. Bosco followed it with low warning rumbles, and Lilly watched the empty spaces with unnerving patience.

The house felt increasingly aware of their presence. The quiet pooled in the corners and stretched through the ceiling cavities as if something inside the structure were tracking their movements. Christopher noticed the pattern immediately. Diana felt it like pressure behind her ribs. Bosco followed it with low warning rumbles, and Lilly watched the empty spaces with unnerving patience.

The house felt increasingly aware of their presence. The quiet pooled in the corners and stretched through the ceiling cavities as if something inside the structure were tracking their movements. Christopher noticed the pattern immediately. Diana felt it like pressure behind her ribs. Bosco followed it with low warning rumbles, and Lilly watched the empty spaces with unnerving patience.

The house felt increasingly aware of their

presence. The quiet pooled in the corners and stretched through the ceiling cavities as if something inside the structure were tracking their movements. Christopher noticed the pattern immediately. Diana felt it like pressure behind her ribs. Bosco followed it with low warning rumbles, and Lilly watched the empty spaces with unnerving patience.

The house felt increasingly aware of their presence. The quiet pooled in the corners and stretched through the ceiling cavities as if something inside the structure were tracking their movements. Christopher noticed the pattern immediately. Diana felt it like pressure behind her ribs. Bosco followed it with low warning rumbles, and Lilly watched the empty spaces with unnerving patience.

The first time Diana felt it outside the house, she nearly convinced herself it was

her imagination.

Nearly.

Walking back from The Blue Jay, she slowed halfway down Juniper Street.

Something in the rhythm of her footsteps felt… off.

She stopped.

Behind her, the sidewalk remained empty.

But the faint sound of a second step echoed half a beat late.

Christopher's warnings came back hard in her memory.

When she reached her front door, Bosco was already inside, barking sharply at the wall

that connected to the blue house.

Diana didn't sleep that night.

Because for the first time…

The house didn't feel contained anymore.

The house felt increasingly aware of their presence. The quiet pooled in the corners and stretched through the ceiling cavities as if something inside the structure were tracking their movements. Christopher noticed the pattern immediately. Diana felt it like pressure behind her ribs. Bosco followed it with low warning rumbles, and Lilly watched the empty spaces

with unnerving patience.

The house felt increasingly aware of their presence. The quiet pooled in the corners and stretched through the ceiling cavities as if something inside the structure were tracking their movements. Christopher noticed the pattern immediately. Diana felt it like pressure behind her ribs. Bosco followed it with low warning rumbles, and Lilly watched the empty spaces with unnerving patience.

The house felt increasingly aware of their presence. The quiet pooled in the corners and stretched through the ceiling cavities as if something inside the structure were tracking their movements. Christopher noticed the pattern immediately. Diana felt it like pressure behind her ribs. Bosco followed it with low warning rumbles, and Lilly watched the empty spaces with unnerving patience.

The house felt increasingly aware of their presence. The quiet pooled in the corners and stretched through the ceiling cavities as if something inside the structure were tracking their movements. Christopher noticed the pattern

immediately. Diana felt it like pressure behind her ribs. Bosco followed it with low warning rumbles, and Lilly watched the empty spaces with unnerving patience.

The house felt increasingly aware of their presence. The quiet pooled in the corners and stretched through the ceiling cavities as if something inside the structure were tracking their movements. Christopher noticed the pattern immediately. Diana felt it like pressure behind her ribs. Bosco followed it with low warning rumbles, and Lilly watched the empty spaces with unnerving patience.

The house felt increasingly aware of their presence. The quiet pooled in the corners and stretched through the ceiling cavities as if something inside the structure were tracking their movements. Christopher noticed the pattern immediately. Diana felt it like pressure behind her ribs. Bosco followed it with low warning rumbles, and Lilly watched the empty spaces with unnerving patience.

The house felt increasingly aware of their presence. The quiet pooled in the corners and

stretched through the ceiling cavities as if something inside the structure were tracking their movements. Christopher noticed the pattern immediately. Diana felt it like pressure behind her ribs. Bosco followed it with low warning rumbles, and Lilly watched the empty spaces with unnerving patience.

The house felt increasingly aware of their presence. The quiet pooled in the corners and stretched through the ceiling cavities as if something inside the structure were tracking their movements. Christopher noticed the pattern immediately. Diana felt it like pressure behind her ribs. Bosco followed it with low warning rumbles, and Lilly watched the empty spaces with unnerving patience.

The house felt increasingly aware of their presence. The quiet pooled in the corners and stretched through the ceiling cavities as if something inside the structure were tracking their movements. Christopher noticed the pattern immediately. Diana felt it like pressure behind her ribs. Bosco followed it with low warning rumbles, and Lilly watched the empty spaces with unnerving patience.

The house felt increasingly aware of their presence. The quiet pooled in the corners and stretched through the ceiling cavities as if something inside the structure were tracking their movements. Christopher noticed the pattern immediately. Diana felt it like pressure behind her ribs. Bosco followed it with low warning rumbles, and Lilly watched the empty spaces with unnerving patience.

The house felt increasingly aware of their presence. The quiet pooled in the corners and stretched through the ceiling cavities as if something inside the structure were tracking their movements. Christopher noticed the pattern immediately. Diana felt it like pressure behind her ribs. Bosco followed it with low warning rumbles, and Lilly watched the empty spaces with unnerving patience.

The house felt increasingly aware of their presence. The quiet pooled in the corners and stretched through the ceiling cavities as if something inside the structure were tracking their movements. Christopher noticed the pattern immediately. Diana felt it like pressure behind her ribs. Bosco followed it with low warning rumbles, and Lilly watched the empty spaces

with unnerving patience.

The house felt increasingly aware of their presence. The quiet pooled in the corners and stretched through the ceiling cavities as if something inside the structure were tracking their movements. Christopher noticed the pattern immediately. Diana felt it like pressure behind her ribs. Bosco followed it with low warning rumbles, and Lilly watched the empty spaces with unnerving patience.

The house felt increasingly aware of their presence. The quiet pooled in the corners and stretched through the ceiling cavities as if something inside the structure were tracking their movements. Christopher noticed the pattern immediately. Diana felt it like pressure behind her ribs. Bosco followed it with low warning rumbles, and Lilly watched the empty spaces with unnerving patience.

The house felt increasingly aware of their presence. The quiet pooled in the corners and stretched through the ceiling cavities as if something inside the structure were tracking their movements. Christopher noticed the pattern

immediately. Diana felt it like pressure behind her ribs. Bosco followed it with low warning rumbles, and Lilly watched the empty spaces with unnerving patience.

The house felt increasingly aware of their presence. The quiet pooled in the corners and stretched through the ceiling cavities as if something inside the structure were tracking their movements. Christopher noticed the pattern immediately. Diana felt it like pressure behind her ribs. Bosco followed it with low warning rumbles, and Lilly watched the empty spaces with unnerving patience.

The house felt increasingly aware of their presence. The quiet pooled in the corners and stretched through the ceiling cavities as if something inside the structure were tracking their movements. Christopher noticed the pattern immediately. Diana felt it like pressure behind her ribs. Bosco followed it with low warning rumbles, and Lilly watched the empty spaces with unnerving patience.

Christopher worked through the night mapping the newly discovered overlaps between the blue house

and the neighboring structures. By 2:30 a.m., the pattern was undeniable.

The hidden cavities formed a continuous path.

Not random renovations.

Not sloppy additions.

A route.

Diana stood behind him, arms wrapped tight around herself. "You're saying something could move

between the houses without ever being seen?"

Christopher didn't look up.

"I'm saying," he replied quietly, "that someone designed it that way."

From inside the shared wall… something shifted slowly in response.

The structure of the house felt increasingly intentional. The quiet did not simply exist anymore; it gathered and shifted as if something within the walls were tracking their movements in real time. Christopher noticed the pattern immediately. Diana felt it like pressure behind her ribs. Bosco followed it with low warning rumbles, and Lilly watched the empty spaces with unnerving patience.

The structure of the house felt increasingly intentional. The quiet did not simply exist anymore; it gathered and shifted as if something within the walls were tracking their movements in real time. Christopher noticed the pattern immediately. Diana felt it like pressure behind her ribs. Bosco followed it with low warning rum-

bles, and Lilly watched the empty spaces with unnerving patience.

The structure of the house felt increasingly intentional. The quiet did not simply exist anymore; it gathered and shifted as if something within the walls were tracking their movements in real time. Christopher noticed the pattern immediately. Diana felt it like pressure behind her ribs. Bosco followed it with low warning rumbles, and Lilly watched the empty spaces with unnerving patience.

The structure of the house felt increasingly intentional. The quiet did not simply exist anymore; it gathered and shifted as if something within the walls were tracking their movements in real time. Christopher noticed the pattern immediately. Diana felt it like pressure behind her ribs. Bosco followed it with low warning rumbles, and Lilly watched the empty spaces with unnerving patience.

The structure of the house felt increasingly intentional. The quiet did not simply exist anymore; it gathered and shifted as if something within the walls were tracking their movements

in real time. Christopher noticed the pattern immediately. Diana felt it like pressure behind her ribs. Bosco followed it with low warning rumbles, and Lilly watched the empty spaces with unnerving patience.

The structure of the house felt increasingly intentional. The quiet did not simply exist anymore; it gathered and shifted as if something within the walls were tracking their movements in real time. Christopher noticed the pattern immediately. Diana felt it like pressure behind her ribs. Bosco followed it with low warning rumbles, and Lilly watched the empty spaces with unnerving patience.

The structure of the house felt increasingly intentional. The quiet did not simply exist anymore; it gathered and shifted as if something within the walls were tracking their movements in real time. Christopher noticed the pattern immediately. Diana felt it like pressure behind her ribs. Bosco followed it with low warning rumbles, and Lilly watched the empty spaces with unnerving patience.

The structure of the house felt increasing-

ly intentional. The quiet did not simply exist anymore; it gathered and shifted as if something within the walls were tracking their movements in real time. Christopher noticed the pattern immediately. Diana felt it like pressure behind her ribs. Bosco followed it with low warning rumbles, and Lilly watched the empty spaces with unnerving patience.

The structure of the house felt increasingly intentional. The quiet did not simply exist anymore; it gathered and shifted as if something within the walls were tracking their movements in real time. Christopher noticed the pattern immediately. Diana felt it like pressure behind her ribs. Bosco followed it with low warning rumbles, and Lilly watched the empty spaces with unnerving patience.

The structure of the house felt increasingly intentional. The quiet did not simply exist anymore; it gathered and shifted as if something within the walls were tracking their movements in real time. Christopher noticed the pattern immediately. Diana felt it like pressure behind her ribs. Bosco followed it with low warning rumbles, and Lilly watched the empty spaces with unnerving patience.

The structure of the house felt increasingly intentional. The quiet did not simply exist anymore; it gathered and shifted as if something within the walls were tracking their movements in real time. Christopher noticed the pattern immediately. Diana felt it like pressure behind her ribs. Bosco followed it with low warning rumbles, and Lilly watched the empty spaces with unnerving patience.

The structure of the house felt increasingly intentional. The quiet did not simply exist anymore; it gathered and shifted as if something within the walls were tracking their movements in real time. Christopher noticed the pattern immediately. Diana felt it like pressure behind her ribs. Bosco followed it with low warning rumbles, and Lilly watched the empty spaces with unnerving patience.

The structure of the house felt increasingly intentional. The quiet did not simply exist anymore; it gathered and shifted as if something within the walls were tracking their movements in real time. Christopher noticed the pattern immediately. Diana felt it like pressure behind her ribs. Bosco followed it with low warning rum-

bles, and Lilly watched the empty spaces with unnerving patience.

The structure of the house felt increasingly intentional. The quiet did not simply exist anymore; it gathered and shifted as if something within the walls were tracking their movements in real time. Christopher noticed the pattern immediately. Diana felt it like pressure behind her ribs. Bosco followed it with low warning rumbles, and Lilly watched the empty spaces with unnerving patience.

The structure of the house felt increasingly intentional. The quiet did not simply exist anymore; it gathered and shifted as if something within the walls were tracking their movements in real time. Christopher noticed the pattern immediately. Diana felt it like pressure behind her ribs. Bosco followed it with low warning rumbles, and Lilly watched the empty spaces with unnerving patience.

The structure of the house felt increasingly intentional. The quiet did not simply exist anymore; it gathered and shifted as if something within the walls were tracking their movements

in real time. Christopher noticed the pattern immediately. Diana felt it like pressure behind her
ribs. Bosco followed it with low warning rumbles, and Lilly watched the empty spaces with
unnerving patience.

The structure of the house felt increasingly intentional. The quiet did not simply exist
anymore; it gathered and shifted as if something
within the walls were tracking their movements
in real time. Christopher noticed the pattern immediately. Diana felt it like pressure behind her
ribs. Bosco followed it with low warning rumbles, and Lilly watched the empty spaces with
unnerving patience.

The city archives did not help.

Christopher pulled every permit record tied to the Keller property, but the older filings were incomplete — sections missing, revisions un-signed.

One blueprint in particular made his pulse jump.

It showed only the original house footprint.

No secondary framing.

No interior channels.

Lenny leaned over the table and tapped the paper once.

"That's not an oversight," he said softly. "That's a removal."

Diana felt cold settle into her bones.

Because if the plans had been altered deliberately…

Someone had been protecting the secret for decades.

The structure of the house felt increasingly intentional. The quiet did not simply exist anymore; it gathered and shifted as if something within the walls were tracking their movements in real time. Christopher noticed the pattern immediately. Diana felt it like pressure behind her ribs. Bosco followed it with low warning rumbles, and Lilly watched the empty spaces with unnerving patience.

The structure of the house felt increasingly intentional. The quiet did not simply exist anymore; it gathered and shifted as if something within the walls were tracking their movements in real time. Christopher noticed the pattern immediately. Diana felt it like pressure behind her ribs. Bosco followed it with low warning rumbles, and Lilly watched the empty spaces with unnerving patience.

The structure of the house felt increasingly intentional. The quiet did not simply exist anymore; it gathered and shifted as if something within the walls were tracking their movements in real time. Christopher noticed the pattern immediately. Diana felt it like pressure behind her ribs. Bosco followed it with low warning rumbles, and Lilly watched the empty spaces with unnerving patience.

The structure of the house felt increasingly intentional. The quiet did not simply exist anymore; it gathered and shifted as if something within the walls were tracking their movements in real time. Christopher noticed the pattern immediately. Diana felt it like pressure behind her ribs. Bosco followed it with low warning rumbles, and Lilly watched the empty spaces with unnerving patience.

The structure of the house felt increasingly intentional. The quiet did not simply exist anymore; it gathered and shifted as if something within the walls were tracking their movements in real time. Christopher noticed the pattern immediately. Diana felt it like pressure behind her ribs. Bosco followed it with low warning rumbles, and Lilly watched the empty spaces with unnerving patience.

The structure of the house felt increasingly intentional. The quiet did not simply exist anymore; it gathered and shifted as if something within the walls were tracking their movements in real time. Christopher noticed the pattern immediately. Diana felt it like pressure behind her ribs. Bosco followed it with low warning rumbles, and Lilly watched the empty spaces with unnerving patience.

The structure of the house felt increasingly intentional. The quiet did not simply exist anymore; it gathered and shifted as if something within the walls were tracking their movements in real time. Christopher noticed the pattern immediately. Diana felt it like pressure behind her ribs. Bosco followed it with low warning rumbles, and Lilly watched the empty spaces with

unnerving patience.

The structure of the house felt increasingly intentional. The quiet did not simply exist
anymore; it gathered and shifted as if something
within the walls were tracking their movements
in real time. Christopher noticed the pattern immediately. Diana felt it like pressure behind her
ribs. Bosco followed it with low warning rumbles, and Lilly watched the empty spaces with
unnerving patience.

The structure of the house felt increasingly intentional. The quiet did not simply exist
anymore; it gathered and shifted as if something
within the walls were tracking their movements
in real time. Christopher noticed the pattern immediately. Diana felt it like pressure behind her
ribs. Bosco followed it with low warning rumbles, and Lilly watched the empty spaces with
unnerving patience.

The structure of the house felt increasingly intentional. The quiet did not simply exist
anymore; it gathered and shifted as if something
within the walls were tracking their movements
in real time. Christopher noticed the pattern im-

mediately. Diana felt it like pressure behind her ribs. Bosco followed it with low warning rumbles, and Lilly watched the empty spaces with unnerving patience.

The structure of the house felt increasingly intentional. The quiet did not simply exist anymore; it gathered and shifted as if something within the walls were tracking their movements in real time. Christopher noticed the pattern immediately. Diana felt it like pressure behind her ribs. Bosco followed it with low warning rumbles, and Lilly watched the empty spaces with unnerving patience.

The structure of the house felt increasingly intentional. The quiet did not simply exist anymore; it gathered and shifted as if something within the walls were tracking their movements in real time. Christopher noticed the pattern immediately. Diana felt it like pressure behind her ribs. Bosco followed it with low warning rumbles, and Lilly watched the empty spaces with unnerving patience.

The structure of the house felt increasingly intentional. The quiet did not simply exist anymore; it gathered and shifted as if something within the walls were tracking their movements in real time. Christopher noticed the pattern immediately. Diana felt it like pressure behind her ribs. Bosco followed it with low warning rumbles, and Lilly watched the empty spaces with unnerving patience.

The structure of the house felt increasingly intentional. The quiet did not simply exist anymore; it gathered and shifted as if something within the walls were tracking their movements in real time. Christopher noticed the pattern immediately. Diana felt it like pressure behind her ribs. Bosco followed it with low warning rumbles, and Lilly watched the empty spaces with unnerving patience.

The structure of the house felt increasingly intentional. The quiet did not simply exist anymore; it gathered and shifted as if something within the walls were tracking their movements in real time. Christopher noticed the pattern immediately. Diana felt it like pressure behind her ribs. Bosco followed it with low warning rumbles, and Lilly watched the empty spaces with unnerving patience.

The structure of the house felt increasingly intentional. The quiet did not simply exist anymore; it gathered and shifted as if something within the walls were tracking their movements in real time. Christopher noticed the pattern immediately. Diana felt it like pressure behind her ribs. Bosco followed it with low warning rumbles, and Lilly watched the empty spaces with unnerving patience.

The structure of the house felt increasingly intentional. The quiet did not simply exist anymore; it gathered and shifted as if something within the walls were tracking their movements in real time. Christopher noticed the pattern immediately. Diana felt it like pressure behind her ribs. Bosco followed it with low warning rumbles, and Lilly watched the empty spaces with unnerving patience.

Diana cornered Lenny the following evening.

For the first time since she had met him, he looked genuinely tired.

"You knew more," she said quietly.

Lenny exhaled slowly and rubbed his face. "Back in '65… there were complaints before Keller

vanished. People heard movement where there shouldn't have been any."

Christopher's voice tightened. "Inside the walls."

Lenny nodded once.

"But the reports never stuck. Too strange. Too easy to dismiss."

Outside, Bosco began barking sharply at the shared property line.

Lilly's head snapped toward the same wall.

Because something had just passed through again.

The structure of the house felt increasingly intentional. The quiet did not simply exist anymore; it gathered and shifted as if something within the walls were tracking their movements in real time. Christopher noticed the pattern immediately. Diana felt it like pressure behind her ribs. Bosco followed it with low warning rumbles, and Lilly watched the empty spaces with unnerving patience.

The structure of the house felt increasingly intentional. The quiet did not simply exist anymore; it gathered and shifted as if something within the walls were tracking their movements in real time. Christopher noticed the pattern immediately. Diana felt it like pressure behind her ribs. Bosco followed it with low warning rumbles, and Lilly watched the empty spaces with unnerving patience.

The structure of the house felt increasingly intentional. The quiet did not simply exist anymore; it gathered and shifted as if something within the walls were tracking their movements in real time. Christopher noticed the pattern immediately. Diana felt it like pressure behind her ribs. Bosco followed it with low warning rumbles, and Lilly watched the empty spaces with unnerving patience.

The structure of the house felt increasingly intentional. The quiet did not simply exist anymore; it gathered and shifted as if something within the walls were tracking their movements in real time. Christopher noticed the pattern immediately. Diana felt it like pressure behind her ribs. Bosco followed it with low warning rumbles, and Lilly watched the empty spaces with unnerving patience.

The structure of the house felt increasingly intentional. The quiet did not simply exist anymore; it gathered and shifted as if something within the walls were tracking their movements in real time. Christopher noticed the pattern immediately. Diana felt it like pressure behind her ribs. Bosco followed it with low warning rumbles, and Lilly watched the empty spaces with unnerving patience.

The structure of the house felt increasingly intentional. The quiet did not simply exist anymore; it gathered and shifted as if something within the walls were tracking their movements in real time. Christopher noticed the pattern immediately. Diana felt it like pressure behind her ribs. Bosco followed it with low warning rumbles, and Lilly watched the empty spaces with unnerving patience.

The structure of the house felt increasingly intentional. The quiet did not simply exist anymore; it gathered and shifted as if something within the walls were tracking their movements in real time. Christopher noticed the pattern immediately. Diana felt it like pressure behind her ribs. Bosco followed it with low warning rumbles, and Lilly watched the empty spaces with unnerving patience.

The structure of the house felt increasingly intentional. The quiet did not simply exist anymore; it gathered and shifted as if something within the walls were tracking their movements in real time. Christopher noticed the pattern immediately. Diana felt it like pressure behind her ribs. Bosco followed it with low warning rumbles, and Lilly watched the empty spaces with unnerving patience.

The structure of the house felt increasingly intentional. The quiet did not simply exist anymore; it gathered and shifted as if something within the walls were tracking their movements in real time. Christopher noticed the pattern immediately. Diana felt it like pressure behind her ribs. Bosco followed it with low warning rumbles, and Lilly watched the empty spaces with unnerving patience.

The structure of the house felt increasingly intentional. The quiet did not simply exist anymore; it gathered and shifted as if something within the walls were tracking their movements in real time. Christopher noticed the pattern immediately. Diana felt it like pressure behind her ribs. Bosco followed it with low warning rumbles, and Lilly watched the empty spaces with

unnerving patience.

The structure of the house felt increasingly intentional. The quiet did not simply exist
anymore; it gathered and shifted as if something
within the walls were tracking their movements
in real time. Christopher noticed the pattern immediately. Diana felt it like pressure behind her
ribs. Bosco followed it with low warning rumbles, and Lilly watched the empty spaces with
unnerving patience.

The structure of the house felt increasingly intentional. The quiet did not simply exist
anymore; it gathered and shifted as if something
within the walls were tracking their movements
in real time. Christopher noticed the pattern immediately. Diana felt it like pressure behind her
ribs. Bosco followed it with low warning rumbles, and Lilly watched the empty spaces with
unnerving patience.

The structure of the house felt increasingly intentional. The quiet did not simply exist
anymore; it gathered and shifted as if something
within the walls were tracking their movements
in real time. Christopher noticed the pattern im-

mediately. Diana felt it like pressure behind her ribs. Bosco followed it with low warning rumbles, and Lilly watched the empty spaces with unnerving patience.

The structure of the house felt increasingly intentional. The quiet did not simply exist anymore; it gathered and shifted as if something within the walls were tracking their movements in real time. Christopher noticed the pattern immediately. Diana felt it like pressure behind her ribs. Bosco followed it with low warning rumbles, and Lilly watched the empty spaces with unnerving patience.

The structure of the house felt increasingly intentional. The quiet did not simply exist anymore; it gathered and shifted as if something within the walls were tracking their movements in real time. Christopher noticed the pattern immediately. Diana felt it like pressure behind her ribs. Bosco followed it with low warning rumbles, and Lilly watched the empty spaces with unnerving patience.

The structure of the house felt increasingly intentional. The quiet did not simply exist anymore; it gathered and shifted as if something within the walls were tracking their movements in real time. Christopher noticed the pattern immediately. Diana felt it like pressure behind her ribs. Bosco followed it with low warning rumbles, and Lilly watched the empty spaces with unnerving patience.

The structure of the house felt increasingly intentional. The quiet did not simply exist anymore; it gathered and shifted as if something within the walls were tracking their movements in real time. Christopher noticed the pattern immediately. Diana felt it like pressure behind her ribs. Bosco followed it with low warning rumbles, and Lilly watched the empty spaces with unnerving patience.

The clearest footage came at 3:07 a.m.

Christopher replayed it five times before speaking.

A distortion crossed the upstairs hallway — not fully solid, not fully shadow.

Human height.

Wrong posture.

It moved through the narrow space between two walls that should not have connected.

Diana's breath caught. "That's… that's a person."

Christopher shook his head slowly.

"No," he said. "A person couldn't fit there."

Bosco's growl rose into a sharp bark.

Because the camera timestamp glitched again…

And the shape turned toward the lens.

The structure of the house felt increasingly intentional. The quiet did not simply exist
anymore; it gathered and shifted as if something
within the walls were tracking their movements
in real time. Christopher noticed the pattern immediately. Diana felt it like pressure behind her
ribs. Bosco followed it with low warning rumbles, and Lilly watched the empty spaces with
unnerving patience.

The structure of the house felt increasingly intentional. The quiet did not simply exist
anymore; it gathered and shifted as if something
within the walls were tracking their movements

in real time. Christopher noticed the pattern immediately. Diana felt it like pressure behind her ribs. Bosco followed it with low warning rumbles, and Lilly watched the empty spaces with unnerving patience.

The structure of the house felt increasingly intentional. The quiet did not simply exist anymore; it gathered and shifted as if something within the walls were tracking their movements in real time. Christopher noticed the pattern immediately. Diana felt it like pressure behind her ribs. Bosco followed it with low warning rumbles, and Lilly watched the empty spaces with unnerving patience.

The structure of the house felt increasingly intentional. The quiet did not simply exist anymore; it gathered and shifted as if something within the walls were tracking their movements in real time. Christopher noticed the pattern immediately. Diana felt it like pressure behind her ribs. Bosco followed it with low warning rumbles, and Lilly watched the empty spaces with unnerving patience.

The structure of the house felt increasing-

ly intentional. The quiet did not simply exist anymore; it gathered and shifted as if something within the walls were tracking their movements in real time. Christopher noticed the pattern immediately. Diana felt it like pressure behind her ribs. Bosco followed it with low warning rumbles, and Lilly watched the empty spaces with unnerving patience.

The structure of the house felt increasingly intentional. The quiet did not simply exist anymore; it gathered and shifted as if something within the walls were tracking their movements in real time. Christopher noticed the pattern immediately. Diana felt it like pressure behind her ribs. Bosco followed it with low warning rumbles, and Lilly watched the empty spaces with unnerving patience.

The structure of the house felt increasingly intentional. The quiet did not simply exist anymore; it gathered and shifted as if something within the walls were tracking their movements in real time. Christopher noticed the pattern immediately. Diana felt it like pressure behind her ribs. Bosco followed it with low warning rumbles, and Lilly watched the empty spaces with unnerving patience.

The structure of the house felt increasingly intentional. The quiet did not simply exist
anymore; it gathered and shifted as if something
within the walls were tracking their movements
in real time. Christopher noticed the pattern immediately. Diana felt it like pressure behind her
ribs. Bosco followed it with low warning rumbles, and Lilly watched the empty spaces with
unnerving patience.

The structure of the house felt increasingly intentional. The quiet did not simply exist
anymore; it gathered and shifted as if something
within the walls were tracking their movements
in real time. Christopher noticed the pattern immediately. Diana felt it like pressure behind her
ribs. Bosco followed it with low warning rumbles, and Lilly watched the empty spaces with
unnerving patience.

The structure of the house felt increasingly intentional. The quiet did not simply exist
anymore; it gathered and shifted as if something
within the walls were tracking their movements
in real time. Christopher noticed the pattern immediately. Diana felt it like pressure behind her
ribs. Bosco followed it with low warning rum-

bles, and Lilly watched the empty spaces with unnerving patience.

The structure of the house felt increasingly intentional. The quiet did not simply exist anymore; it gathered and shifted as if something within the walls were tracking their movements in real time. Christopher noticed the pattern immediately. Diana felt it like pressure behind her ribs. Bosco followed it with low warning rumbles, and Lilly watched the empty spaces with unnerving patience.

The structure of the house felt increasingly intentional. The quiet did not simply exist anymore; it gathered and shifted as if something within the walls were tracking their movements in real time. Christopher noticed the pattern immediately. Diana felt it like pressure behind her ribs. Bosco followed it with low warning rumbles, and Lilly watched the empty spaces with unnerving patience.

The structure of the house felt increasingly intentional. The quiet did not simply exist anymore; it gathered and shifted as if something within the walls were tracking their movements

in real time. Christopher noticed the pattern immediately. Diana felt it like pressure behind her
ribs. Bosco followed it with low warning rumbles, and Lilly watched the empty spaces with
unnerving patience.

The structure of the house felt increasingly intentional. The quiet did not simply exist
anymore; it gathered and shifted as if something
within the walls were tracking their movements
in real time. Christopher noticed the pattern immediately. Diana felt it like pressure behind her
ribs. Bosco followed it with low warning rumbles, and Lilly watched the empty spaces with
unnerving patience.

The structure of the house felt increasingly intentional. The quiet did not simply exist
anymore; it gathered and shifted as if something
within the walls were tracking their movements
in real time. Christopher noticed the pattern immediately. Diana felt it like pressure behind her
ribs. Bosco followed it with low warning rumbles, and Lilly watched the empty spaces with
unnerving patience.

The structure of the house felt increasing-

ly intentional. The quiet did not simply exist anymore; it gathered and shifted as if something within the walls were tracking their movements in real time. Christopher noticed the pattern immediately. Diana felt it like pressure behind her ribs. Bosco followed it with low warning rumbles, and Lilly watched the empty spaces with unnerving patience.

The structure of the house felt increasingly intentional. The quiet did not simply exist anymore; it gathered and shifted as if something within the walls were tracking their movements in real time. Christopher noticed the pattern immediately. Diana felt it like pressure behind her ribs. Bosco followed it with low warning rumbles, and Lilly watched the empty spaces with unnerving patience.

The final incident happened just before dawn.

Diana woke to the softest sound imaginable — something brushing lightly along the inside of her

bedroom wall.

She sat up slowly, heart already racing.

Bosco was awake.

Rigid.

Silent.

Lilly stood at the doorway, fur slightly raised, eyes locked on the same section of wall.

Then, very clearly — too clearly to dismiss —

A faint voice whispered from inside the structure.

"…Diana."

Her blood turned to ice.

Across the street, every light in the blue house flickered on at once.

Christopher's phone rang seconds later.

His voice came tight and controlled when she answered.

"Diana," he said, "we need to talk about what we just captured."

She swallowed hard. "What did you see?"

There was a long pause.

Then Christopher spoke the words that would carry them into the final book.

"…it's not just moving through the houses anymore."

The structure of the house felt increasingly intentional. The quiet did not simply exist anymore; it gathered and shifted as if something within the walls were tracking their movements in real time. Christopher noticed the pattern immediately. Diana felt it like pressure behind her ribs. Bosco followed it with low warning rumbles, and Lilly watched the empty spaces with unnerving patience.

The structure of the house felt increasingly intentional. The quiet did not simply exist anymore; it gathered and shifted as if something within the walls were tracking their movements

in real time. Christopher noticed the pattern immediately. Diana felt it like pressure behind her ribs. Bosco followed it with low warning rumbles, and Lilly watched the empty spaces with unnerving patience.

The structure of the house felt increasingly intentional. The quiet did not simply exist anymore; it gathered and shifted as if something within the walls were tracking their movements in real time. Christopher noticed the pattern immediately. Diana felt it like pressure behind her ribs. Bosco followed it with low warning rumbles, and Lilly watched the empty spaces with unnerving patience.

The structure of the house felt increasingly intentional. The quiet did not simply exist anymore; it gathered and shifted as if something within the walls were tracking their movements in real time. Christopher noticed the pattern immediately. Diana felt it like pressure behind her ribs. Bosco followed it with low warning rumbles, and Lilly watched the empty spaces with unnerving patience.

The structure of the house felt increasing-

ly intentional. The quiet did not simply exist anymore; it gathered and shifted as if something within the walls were tracking their movements in real time. Christopher noticed the pattern immediately. Diana felt it like pressure behind her ribs. Bosco followed it with low warning rumbles, and Lilly watched the empty spaces with unnerving patience.

The structure of the house felt increasingly intentional. The quiet did not simply exist anymore; it gathered and shifted as if something within the walls were tracking their movements in real time. Christopher noticed the pattern immediately. Diana felt it like pressure behind her ribs. Bosco followed it with low warning rumbles, and Lilly watched the empty spaces with unnerving patience.

The structure of the house felt increasingly intentional. The quiet did not simply exist anymore; it gathered and shifted as if something within the walls were tracking their movements in real time. Christopher noticed the pattern immediately. Diana felt it like pressure behind her ribs. Bosco followed it with low warning rumbles, and Lilly watched the empty spaces with unnerving patience.

The structure of the house felt increasingly intentional. The quiet did not simply exist anymore; it gathered and shifted as if something within the walls were tracking their movements in real time. Christopher noticed the pattern immediately. Diana felt it like pressure behind her ribs. Bosco followed it with low warning rumbles, and Lilly watched the empty spaces with unnerving patience.

The structure of the house felt increasingly intentional. The quiet did not simply exist anymore; it gathered and shifted as if something within the walls were tracking their movements in real time. Christopher noticed the pattern immediately. Diana felt it like pressure behind her ribs. Bosco followed it with low warning rumbles, and Lilly watched the empty spaces with unnerving patience.

The structure of the house felt increasingly intentional. The quiet did not simply exist anymore; it gathered and shifted as if something within the walls were tracking their movements in real time. Christopher noticed the pattern immediately. Diana felt it like pressure behind her ribs. Bosco followed it with low warning rum-

bles, and Lilly watched the empty spaces with unnerving patience.

The structure of the house felt increasingly intentional. The quiet did not simply exist anymore; it gathered and shifted as if something within the walls were tracking their movements in real time. Christopher noticed the pattern immediately. Diana felt it like pressure behind her ribs. Bosco followed it with low warning rumbles, and Lilly watched the empty spaces with unnerving patience.

The structure of the house felt increasingly intentional. The quiet did not simply exist anymore; it gathered and shifted as if something within the walls were tracking their movements in real time. Christopher noticed the pattern immediately. Diana felt it like pressure behind her ribs. Bosco followed it with low warning rumbles, and Lilly watched the empty spaces with unnerving patience.

The structure of the house felt increasingly intentional. The quiet did not simply exist anymore; it gathered and shifted as if something within the walls were tracking their movements

in real time. Christopher noticed the pattern immediately. Diana felt it like pressure behind her
ribs. Bosco followed it with low warning rumbles, and Lilly watched the empty spaces with
unnerving patience.

The structure of the house felt increasingly intentional. The quiet did not simply exist
anymore; it gathered and shifted as if something
within the walls were tracking their movements
in real time. Christopher noticed the pattern immediately. Diana felt it like pressure behind her
ribs. Bosco followed it with low warning rumbles, and Lilly watched the empty spaces with
unnerving patience.

The structure of the house felt increasingly intentional. The quiet did not simply exist
anymore; it gathered and shifted as if something
within the walls were tracking their movements
in real time. Christopher noticed the pattern immediately. Diana felt it like pressure behind her
ribs. Bosco followed it with low warning rumbles, and Lilly watched the empty spaces with
unnerving patience.

The structure of the house felt increasing-

ly intentional. The quiet did not simply exist anymore; it gathered and shifted as if something within the walls were tracking their movements in real time. Christopher noticed the pattern immediately. Diana felt it like pressure behind her ribs. Bosco followed it with low warning rumbles, and Lilly watched the empty spaces with unnerving patience.

If Book One made you uneasy, Book Two pulls you deeper.

The strange events inside the house were only the beginning. As Christopher begins taking a more active role in uncovering the truth, the pattern behind the disturbances becomes impossible to ignore. What once felt like coincidence now points to something deliberate — and far more dangerous.

In Book Two, the stakes escalate:

The house begins to reveal its history

Christopher shifts from reacting to investigating

Bosco and Lilly's behavior becomes critically important

The threat proves it is very real

Readers who love layered suspense will appreciate how the mystery widens while the tension tightens. Questions from Book One don't just get answers — they open doors that may have been better left closed.

About the Author — Robert Armstrong

Robert Armstrong is a prolific creative storyteller, illustrator, and independent publisher dedicated to building immersive reading experiences across multiple genres. As the driving force behind numerous publishing projects, Armstrong combines suspenseful fiction, interactive puzzle books, motivational journals, and imaginative children's titles into a growing body of work designed to engage readers of all ages.

With a strong focus on emotional resonance and reader engagement, Armstrong's fiction—particularly The Quiet House series—blends domestic suspense with psychological tension, creating stories that linger long after the final page. His work often features carefully developed characters, layered mysteries, and meaningful emotional threads that reward attentive readers.

Beyond thrillers, Armstrong is widely recognized for creating interactive and uplifting content through brands such as Library User Group and related creative imprints. His publishing catalog spans coloring adventures, humor collections, resilience-focused journals, and forward-looking explorations of technology and society. This cross-genre versatility reflects his core mission: to inspire curiosity, creativity, and personal growth through accessible, engaging books.

Armstrong approaches each project with an entrepreneurial spirit and a hands-on creative process, emphasizing high-quality design, consistent visual identity, and reader-focused storytelling. Whether crafting suspense that keeps readers turning pages late into the night or developing family-friendly interactive books, his goal remains the same — to create experiences that entertain, encourage, and connect.

www.ingramcontent.com/pod-product-compliance
Lightning Source LLC
Chambersburg PA
CBHW061503050726

47593CB00002B/427